Boundless Blessings and God's Grace

My Journey through Breast Cancer

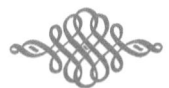

Cynthia J. Eggl

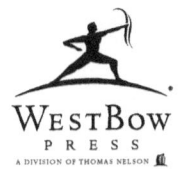

WestBow
PRESS
A DIVISION OF THOMAS NELSON

WestBow Press books may be ordered through booksellers or by contacting:

WestBow Press
A Division of Thomas Nelson
1663 Liberty Drive
Bloomington, IN 47403
www.westbowpress.com
1-(866) 928-1240

ISBN: 978-1-4497-7813-2 (e)
ISBN: 978-1-4497-7812-5 (sc)
ISBN: 978-1-4497-7811-8 (hc)

Library of Congress Control Number: 2012922792

Printed in the United States of America

WestBow Press rev. date: 12/07/2012

*To God, who has seen me through this journey and
blessed me beyond measure in my life.*

▼

Foreword

On April 12, 2011, I was diagnosed with breast cancer. To say I was in shock is a huge understatement. We did not have a breast cancer history on either my mother's or father's side of the family. My brother, Fred, had waged a valiant battle with brain cancer when he was diagnosed at the age of 17. He passed away at the age of 21. He faced his battle with courage and determination, and could not have been braver. So after one of my siblings had already lost a battle with cancer, was this really happening to me?

I have not always been an outgoing person. As a little girl, I was quite shy. But as I grew older, I started to enjoy meeting people, those I already knew and new people. It was an opportunity to help make their day a better day for having seen, met, and talked with me. I also felt it was important for me to smile not only with my mouth but also with my eyes.

I still live my life like that now, but now I also take every opportunity afforded me to talk with people, both women and men, about the importance of monthly self-breast exams, mammograms, annual physical exams, and just plainly to know your own body. If there are changes or pain in your body, do not hesitate to schedule a checkup because, the sooner you identify and get a diagnosis, especially if it is breast cancer or any other form of cancer, the better your chances of survival, and your treatments, surgery, recovery, and healing will be less traumatic. I also inform women that one in eight of us will be diagnosed with breast cancer. And men, this is not only a women's disease. Five percent of men get breast cancer, too.

Being able to reach out and help others going through a similar experience has brought great meaning to my life, especially since my diagnosis. Reaching out to touch their arm in support, smiling, and asking them to fight with everything they are, reassuring them that God is by their side, along with a tremendous medical team and many people praying and caring for them and loving them have been a blessing to me. One prayerful passage and one quote has stuck with me through my breast cancer journey.

> *I have spread my wings of faith to embrace the "Wind," placing my heart in Jesus. I have experienced quiet, "everyday" miracles. His joy has balanced my pain, his power has lifted my burden, his peace has calmed my worries, his grace has been more than adequate to cover me, his strength has been sufficient to carry me through, and his love has bathed my wounds like a healing balm.* Excerpt from "Why? Trusting God When You Don't Understand" by Anne Graham Lotz.

This passage sums up my feelings about how my breast cancer battle unfolded and my successful recovery to date. I printed the following quote and placed it on my dresser in my bedroom, and I read it every morning and night: *"You never know how strong you are, until being strong is the only choice you have"* (Author Unknown).

I can emphatically say that I am a better person for having gone through this battle, and I can only pray that God sees fit to continue to let me share my journey with others for many years to come, just as many survivors and family members of those who have lost their battles did to encourage me along.

This journey has reminded me to never take anything for granted, to be grateful for every day I am on the face of the Earth, and to make the most of each day. Within each of us are a fighting spirit and, hopefully, a recognition that we are not in total control of our lives. God is, and he will determine when, where, and how we will pass from this world. Until then, we need to accept the difficulties that we encounter in our lives with dignity, grace, determination, and knowing that he is constantly by our side. I try to remember that, through God's blessings and all of the countless prayers, compassion, care, and love, I am here to continue to live my life, working to be a healthier person so I can do the work that God has entrusted me to accomplish.

Acknowledgments

To my mother, Jan, and my sister Jill, my primary caregivers throughout my breast cancer battle, I will be forever indebted to you for your steadfast love, diligent care, and constant support and prayers.

To my sister Vicki and her husband, Tom; my brother Mark and his wife, Carla Ann; and to my brother Scott and his wife, Kathy, I don't know how to thank you enough for your prayerful vigilance, love, humor, and stoicism, which made me strong when this diagnosis rocked my world. You all remain firmly planted in my heart.

To my nieces, Melissa, Betsy, and Ashley, and my nephew, Stephen, I felt your presence, strength, and love every day of this journey. How much more blessed could I be. Thank you.

I am fortunate to have a large family of aunts and uncles and many cousins and their spouses who shared knowledge and reached out to prayer chains to make certain I was being lifted up and carried along the way. I am certain that everyone who goes through this type of ordeal feels that his or her family is special. I know mine is extraordinary.

There is just simply not a way that seems adequate enough to thank the many friends, coworkers, colleagues, business acquaintances, churches, prayer chains, my Cando connections, and, no doubt, people I am not even aware of who, along with God, have carried me through this life-altering phase of my life with compassion and prayer. The kindnesses shown to my family and me through this battle have reaffirmed that goodness is truly in the world, and it has surrounded me and lifted me up with each step of this journey. Thank you.

Finally, to the tremendous team of medical professionals at Sanford Health's Roger Maris Cancer Center and throughout their health system, your skillful care and compassionate dedication to me as a patient has enriched my life and, quite literally, saved it. "Thank you" really does seem woefully inadequate, but know my thanks come straight from my heart and I will be forever grateful for your outstanding care.

Boundless blessings and God's grace have carried me through the battle of my life. Love you all!

DIAGNOSIS

Wednesday, April 13, 2011, 5:00 p.m., CDT

The Battle Begins

I wanted to let you know that I had biopsies done on Monday on my left breast and one lymph node, and all three areas came back yesterday afternoon, April 12, 2011, indicating I have breast cancer. The two tumors are located in the lower portion of the left breast, one that is four centimeters and a slightly smaller one below that one. A lymph node tested positive for breast cancer in the same region near the tumors. Just to reiterate, I had my first baseline mammogram when I was thirty-five, and starting at forty, I have had a yearly mammogram, including one last May, which was clear. I do have very dense breast tissue, and because of weight training and additional muscle that builds, it has been very difficult for them to read any of my scans. It was also difficult for me to feel any lump until a week ago Monday, April 4, 2011. As soon as I felt a lump, I called to schedule an appointment, and Sanford Health's Roger Maris Cancer Center has moved me through the system as quickly as possible. My oncologists and breast surgeon feel I may be battling a fairly aggressive form of cancer that may have been growing for two to four years.

So I will start with a PET scan at the cancer center at 7:30 a.m. this Friday morning to see if cancer affects any other organs or tissues. Positron emission tomography (PET) is a test that uses a special type of camera and a tracer (radioactive chemical) to look at organs in the body. The tracer usually is a special form of a substance (such as glucose) that collects in cells that are using a lot of energy, such as cancer cells.

During the test, the tracer liquid is put into a vein (intravenous, or IV) in your arm. The tracer moves through your body, where much of it

1

collects in the specific organ or tissue. The tracer gives off tiny positively charged particles (positrons). The camera records the positrons and turns the recording into pictures on a computer.

PET scan pictures do not show as much detail as computed tomography (CT) scans or magnetic resonance imaging (MRI) because the pictures show only the location of the tracer. The PET picture may be matched with those from a CT scan to get more detailed information about where the tracer is located.

A PET scan is often used to evaluate cancer, check blood flow, or see how organs are working. For my test, it will be used to determine where the cancer has occurred in my body. Just prior to the PET scan, I will be placed in a dark, quiet room, where the injection is administered, and will lie quietly for an hour. I will then transition into the scanner where the test will be completed.

My first appointment with an oncologist will be Friday at 1:00 p.m., and he will have the results of the PET scan to share at that time. I have an appointment with a radiation oncologist at 2:30 p.m. on Friday to determine how to move forward with the breast surgery, chemo, and radiation treatments based on tests that are being run on the additional tissue that was taken during the biopsies and what my medical team finds in the PET scan. I also have an appointment scheduled with a breast surgeon for Tuesday, April 19, at 9:00 a.m. to schedule surgery.

I am trying to stay positive and brave. Sometimes God makes you walk through a battle such as this. I will fight for the best outcome. I sincerely appreciate your prayers and those of your family and others. Thank you!

A special thank you to my dear friend, Amanda, who drove me to and from my biopsies procedure and stayed with me until Jill, my sister, was able to make it home following my appointment. And to Pat, our family friend from Cando, who came to sit with me while I recovered from the needle biopsies and was with me when I received the call that I had breast cancer – thank you for being so calm and reassuring. I am blessed to have you both in my life!

Friday, April 15, 2011, 7:00 p.m., CDT

Plan of Action

The following update contains quite a bit of information but hopefully provides an adequate explanation of my plan of action to battle my breast cancer intensively for the next nine-plus months and diligently for the rest of my life.

I am relieved to report that results from my PET scan indicated that my breast cancer had not spread to other organs and/or tissue. I gave my medical oncologist, Dr. Amit Panwalkar, a high five for that great news. I do have stage II breast cancer with both tumor types being infiltrating ductal and a tumor grade of III of III carcinoma. The lymph node showed metastatic, high-grade carcinoma. Additional tests of the tumors and lymph node breast cancer indicated that:

- The estrogen receptor assay was positive (which the oncologists said was good news)

- The HER-2/neu was 1+ negative (which the oncologists felt was good news)

- The progesterone receptor assay was negative (which was not such good news)

Both oncologists indicated I was battling a fairly aggressive breast cancer, but it's curable, a huge relief for me. An MRI is scheduled to help provide the breast surgeon with the best information possible for surgery to be performed as soon as possible. The oncologists felt that starting chemo before surgery would not have a huge effect in shrinking the tumors, and because I have two tumors, with tissue to be removed in between, it was felt I should proceed with surgery as soon as possible.

After consulting with my family and reading about the options, I agreed.

There was no indication of affected lymph nodes behind the breastbone or that cancer had compromised the chest wall at this time. The surgeon will perform a lumpectomy on the two tumors and affected tissue area, which could become a mastectomy if the cancerous tissue is more prevalent once the doctor can look at the involved area during surgery. Additionally, the surgeon will remove both level 1 and level 2 lymph nodes below the left arm area next to the cancerous tumors, and additional biopsies will be performed on lymph nodes removed to check for further breast cancer.

The recovery time following surgery will be three to four weeks, with my first chemo session scheduled for early June. I will have a port inserted under my skin, near the collarbone, which will remain in place for my chemo sessions and potentially up to two years. The course of chemo discussed as of today includes an eight-week course of two types, followed by a twelve-week course of a third type and finally a five- to six-week course of radiation because of lymph node involvement. Following chemo and radiation, I will take Tamoxifen for up to five years. This treatment plan could change depending on what the surgeon finds when removing the tumors, additional biopsies on the removed lymph nodes, and how well I tolerate chemo and radiation.

After speaking with the two oncologists, I hope I will be able to work part time. However, it was stressed that this all depends on how I do through potential complications from surgery, chemo, radiation, and the possibility of lymph edema following removal of the lymph nodes under the left arm.

Suffice it to say, I have a battle on my hands, which I intend to win, and I would sincerely appreciate your continued prayers. The outpouring of concern and compassion and the countless prayers and well-wishes have been overwhelming. I am blessed to have you all in my life. I know this will be a life-altering experience. I firmly believe that I will successfully complete my journey. If I haven't said it to you before or often enough, I love you. Thank you!

Tuesday, April 19, 2011, 4:00 p.m., CDT

More Detailed Information

This update will probably contain more information than some of you care to read and, for others, the detailed information you have requested. Right now, this is the best way for me to communicate, so thank you for your understanding. For those of you who just want a summary, my surgery is scheduled for May 2 with a double lumpectomy and removal of the level 1 and 2 lymph nodes under the left arm. Recovery will be three to four weeks with chemo and radiation to follow. For those of you, who requested detailed information, please see below.

I want to thank you all again for your kind e-mails, calls, cards, remembrances, and, most especially, prayers. God smiled on me when he placed you in my life, and I thank him every day. I realize some people are not as comfortable as others when I say "I love you," but just know it is important for me at this time in my life to let you know how important you are to me and I cherish the time we have spent together. I will try to keep you updated as I progress forward in this fight. Until I see you next, take care!

Detailed Information

As an update through Tuesday, April 19, I was not able to complete the MRI on Monday afternoon because of the size of my breast tissue and my overall body size. I followed up with Dr. Panwalkar, and he assured me that he felt the cancer had not spread and we could proceed with surgery and chemo utilizing the imaging we currently have in place. He was concerned about having me travel to either Sioux Falls or the Twin Cities to be able to access an MRI that could accommodate me at this time.

I met with Dr. Michael Bouton, my breast surgeon, this morning (Tuesday) at 9:00 a.m. I will have surgery on Monday, May 2. It is longer than I had anticipated waiting, but I can only place my life in God's hands and pray that the cancer will not spread to other organs and I will successfully make it through my surgery on that date. Dr. Bouton indicated that he is still planning for a double lumpectomy and removal of the level 1 and level 2 lymph nodes under the left arm. I will have a drainage tube placed in the area of the removed lymph nodes, which will remain in place for one to three weeks, depending on how well my body handles fluid in that area. The tissue and the tumors removed will be sent to pathology to determine if there is further breast cancer or if additional tissue in the breast needs to be removed because of proximity to the original tumors. If positive, a second surgery will be performed to remove further tissue and another set of pathology reports run, and if they are still not clear, there is a rare potential for a third surgery removing additional tissue.

I will be released from the hospital the day after surgery to my home for recovery. The surgeon indicated I would be off work for at least two weeks following surgery. He did indicate that one out of four patients suffer lymph edema (swelling of the arm), which may or may not go away over time. One out of four has residual pain underneath the arm where lymph nodes are removed. I would sincerely appreciate extra prayers that I don't suffer those complications.

I have been taken off my herbal supplementation, and as of this morning when I met with Dr. Bouton, I was taken off the high-dose aspirin that had been prescribed following a mini-stroke I suffered on October 26, 2010. According to the scales at the medical facilities, I have gained 6.6 pounds since last Friday at 1:00 p.m. Dr. Panwalkar has asked me to weigh myself at home and track the weight variance, and if I continue to rapidly gain weight, he will put me on medication to pull off the extra fluid. He also indicated I could remain on my high-dose aspirin until next Monday, a week prior to my surgery date, which will provide extra protection as a blood thinner to prevent stroke symptoms. That is giving me better peace of mind.

I was feeling fairly defeated early this afternoon, but after speaking directly with Dr. Panwalkar, he refocused me on preparation, monitoring my condition, staying as healthy as possible prior to surgery, and thinking positively. He is proving to be a great leader of my team, and he reassured me he will see me through this battle. Patience will be a virtue right now, which most of you know is not my strong suit; however, I will try to be good.

Friday, April 29, 2011, 10:09 p.m., CDT

Finished My Workweek

I am happy to report that I made it through this entire workweek being focused on positive things and getting my ducks in a row at work before my surgery on Monday, May 2.

I ordered two new wigs from TLC (American Cancer Society), along with several other necessary items to help me in my recovery following surgery, and they arrived on Wednesday. Jill and I had fun trying on the wigs and getting used to the different styles, and our next-door neighbor Donna even got in on the fun.

So on Thursday evening at my monthly appointment, my hairstylist Lacey took the scissors to my hair, which she said she had really wanted to do for several years, and cut it to look like the wig I will wear when my hair starts to fall out, about two to three weeks after chemo begins. I wanted to get used to seeing myself with the new hairstyle. The next hair step will be in about four weeks when I visit Lacey again, and she gets to give me a very short but stylish cut so it won't be so traumatic when it starts to fall out.

My mom is expected back in Fargo tomorrow afternoon ahead of the bad weather and my surgery. I love my family a lot, so it will be a comfort having Mom and Jill with me on Monday.

Our friend Shari is also joining us tomorrow so we can go for a pedicure together. Jill and Shari get to have their toenails painted following all the other wonderful things that happen during a pedicure, but I have been advised that there will be no nail polish for me, at the request of my surgeon and oncologist's offices, so I can be monitored how I am doing through surgery, recovery, and so forth. So I guess I will embrace the natural look for the foreseeable future.

It is amazing what one takes for granted each day, like:

- Driving (which I won't be doing for two weeks following surgery)

- Making plans to attend events (which I will need to decide one day at a time)

- Our health (which is priceless once it is threatened)

I have to remember each day that I am fighting for my life. You gain a whole new perspective on life, family, friends, coworkers, and what is most important for your future.

As I have mentioned in earlier updates, I am grateful for your thoughts and prayers. They make me sleep more soundly each night, and I am confident they will carry me through this battle. Thank you. Love you lots!

Sunday, May 1, 2011, 8:35 p.m., CDT

Final Preparation before Surgery

It has been a busy weekend. Saturday morning started with my first attempt at styling my new haircut and a few final hours working in the morning and early afternoon at the office. My mom arrived from Cando ahead of the blizzard in western and central North Dakota. We had a fun-filled hour at the nail salon for a pedicure and manicure with Jill and Shari. We ate at a local café and enjoyed some sweet potato pancakes and good company before Shari headed back to Grand Forks. I took a short nap, cleaned some of the condo, read the newspaper, and then joined my family for an evening meal at our favorite seafood restaurant.

The hectic pace continued Sunday morning with four loads of laundry and continued cleaning of the condo. I spoke with a former co-worker, Joan, who now lives in North Carolina. About one year ago, she was also diagnosed with breast cancer and has successfully completed treatment. I watched Sunday Mass on TV, wrote and sent out monthly bills, and packed my bag for my hospital stay. I went to our Catholic church where Father Kevin took an hour out of his very busy schedule for me to go through the sacraments of reconciliation, communion, and anointing me in preparation for my surgery tomorrow morning and continuing treatment following surgery. I visited with a number of friends and neighbors throughout the day. I had a family meal at our favorite pie place. I got my truck filled with gas, vacuumed, and washed. I talked with family members in South Carolina and another traveling by bus to Brainerd, Minnesota, by phone. Finally, I took some time to read the Sunday paper and breathe deeply before taking a shower and heading to bed. Mom, Jill, and I will be at Sanford Health by 6:00 a.m. tomorrow in preparation for my surgery.

I have felt such inner strength and peace since my diagnosis, and that is due, in large part, to your continued prayers, good wishes, positive energy, encouraging cards, kind remembrances, and just being incredibly thoughtful and compassionate family, coworkers, and friends. I am truly blessed to have you all in my life. Thank you. Love you lots!

SURGERY

Tuesday, May 3, 2011, 2:03 p.m., CDT

Out of Surgery (Jill)

Jill here, writing to keep all of you updated on Cindy's progress. I am second in command of "Operation Cindy." Mom is first in command at this time until we can return command over to Cindy.

The surgeon indicated, as far as the surgery is concerned, everything went as anticipated. He did not observe anything he did not expect. Cindy, however, cannot seem to keep ahead of the pain at the incision sites. She was scheduled to be released home today, but Dr. Bouton has decided to connect her to a pump so she can begin to administer her own pain medication. We will wait to see if this will allow her to rest in comfort. Mom and I spent the night at the hospital to make certain Cindy felt secure. I think, many times, family is the best pain medication of all, especially if a person is fortunate enough to get the "Loving Mother" high-potency dosage. We are still waiting for the results of the biopsies to make certain the doctor removed all of the cancer during the surgery.

We appreciate all of your prayers, well-wishes, and good vibes. Only the Lord knows how much pain he is shouldering for Cindy at this time to make it bearable for her.

If things go better today, Cindy should be released tomorrow, where she can rest in her own bed. With your continued prayers, she will hopefully write the next entry. Until then, think good thoughts.

Thursday, May 5, 2011, 6:25 a.m., CDT

Moving Up

Since Jill's last update on Tuesday, it has been a battle between my pain and my toughness, and the pain was winning. After two days using a variety of pain medications, Dr. Bouton finally called in the big guns and decided to have me, the patient, choose when to administer the medication using a pump. I am happy to report that I am finally feeling better, and my pain is easing. I hope to be headed for home soon.

There have been several times in my life where I have had to rely on others to help heal me back to more normal health, and this instance has been one of those times. Boy, was it one of those times. Yesterday, I was moved from my first room, a double room with twice as many visitors as patients and three times as many machines. The same holds true for the number of rotating nurses. There were a lot of them. I have since been moved up to another room late yesterday afternoon. It now feels as if we are at a high-class hotel. We even had sleeping accommodations for both Mom and Jill, and I've had the same nurse since I got here, bless her soul.

On my agenda for today is a positive visit from my surgeon, a potential shower, letting Mom and Jill go home to freshen up, some more good food from the cafeteria, and then hopefully the news that I can go home. We will see – all in good time. (By the way, I have gotten much better at the patience thing the last few days.)

That's it for now. I hope to have another positive report for you all soon. Thank you again for your thoughts and prayers. Love you!

POST SURGERY

Friday, May 6, 2011, 9:05 p.m., CDT

And No More Good Ice Cream

At 1:30 p.m. today, Dr. Bouton came to check to see if I was ready to go home. My pain had been under control since I was told to stop being an overachiever with my rehab exercises and knock off the calisthenics. So, I can't move my arm above shoulder height for the next week and a half. Now I'm told after I had been shampooing and styling my own hair.

It has been a long five days waiting for the pain to subside and the pathology reports to come back, but I am happy to let you know that Dr. Bouton told me today before I left the hospital that the pathology reports had come back clear. So that means no additional surgeries at this time. No doubt all of the prayers have been answered.

At 5:30 p.m., I climbed the stairs up to our condo – home at last. My bed feels great to lie in, and it is good to be home, but we have no good ice cream tonight. I'll live.

As always, thanks for all your thoughts, prayers and kind remembrances, and thanks to my Mom and Jill for being there for me.

Tuesday, May 10, 2011, 10:20 a.m., CDT

Another Hurdle Jumped

It has been a relaxed but full three days of rest and closely monitored physical movement since I was released from the hospital on Friday, May 6. Finding ways to sit in chairs where the drain tube was not painful and incisions didn't pull has been challenging. Even finding comfortable ways to lie in the bed, which normally sounds like such a peaceful and serene thing to do, have been difficult. Trust me when I say I have stayed right on schedule with my pain medication. That has pulled me through so far.

I have prayed since being released from the hospital that when I went for my follow-up visit with Dr. Bouton on May 10 that the drain tube placed near the area of the lymph node removal could be taken out.

This morning, Jamie, my dear friend and wife to my boss, Pat, picked up my mom and me and drove us to my appointment at 8:30 a.m. I still can't drive for at least another week and while I am on the prescribed pain medication. Thank you, Jamie!

When I saw Dr. Bouton, he was very pleased with the progress of the surgical sites and noticed that the drainage through the tube had slowed considerably. So it was removed. Yippee! It will be much easier to take a shower, sit in a chair, put my left hand down by my side, and sleep soundly at night. I still have residual pain at both surgical sites and the drain site for the time being, and I still have strict orders that I should not be lifting my arm above shoulder level and getting too carried away with physical activity, but all in all, things are getting better every day.

I have been amazed at the prayers, thoughts, calls, cards, remembrances, e-mails, guestbook entries, not to mention the personal visits from people who mean so much in my life. My prognosis right now seems very good that I will win my battle. I just have to walk the path toward restored health over the next nine-plus months.

My next appointment is on Tuesday, May 17, Jill's fiftieth birthday. It isn't the way we wanted to celebrate this milestone birthday for her, but as she has reassured me, we will have many years ahead of us to celebrate birthdays. I am counting on that so we can celebrate her big birthday in style someday soon!

It is wonderful to still have:

- My hair to style

- Eyebrows to pluck (normally not one of my favorite things, especially when there are fewer to work with and they are getting grayer)

- Eyelashes to apply mascara to

I just generally try to keep myself looking as good as possible on the outside. We take so much for granted on a daily basis. This type of diagnosis truly puts thing into perspective and makes you appreciate all that God has blessed you with in your life. And by having you work with the challenges on the outside, God restores peace, strength, persistence, caring, compassion, and a need to share your journey, both good and bad on the inside, so that when you close your eyes at night or during naps each day, you can rest with a calm and comforted heart and soul.

This caring and compassionate nature holds true when referring to my family; friends; current and former coworkers; classmates; board, committee, and general members at the nonprofit organization where I work; businesspeople who I have encountered and worked with over the years and who have been by my side through good and challenging instances; and inspirational people who God has strategically placed in my life. I may not have recognized it at the time, but it makes total sense now. And those folks just have a strong sense of compassion, reaching out to others in need, and they are gracious enough to share it on a daily basis.

Thank you all for reaching out to my family and me in the manner that makes you feel the most comfortable. Please know that I will never forget your kindnesses and prayers or take it for granted. I am grateful you are all part of my life, and I love you very much. Take care and know that I am hanging in there and taking it one day at a time.

Monday, May 16, 2011, 9:44 a.m., CDT

Getting Ready for the Next Phase

Normally, you will find my journal entries fairly upbeat and written with a sense of humor. However, I had a really rough night last night, and thank God my mom was there by my side. It is very challenging to try to sleep and find a comfortable way to lie where my side does not hurt. My surgeon has told me that it will take time, and being on pain medication for a length of time also takes its toll. I am doing all I can do right now to stay ahead of the pain. My days seem better, but the pain I am feeling never has really gone away since my surgery. I am trying to tolerate it the best I can and be brave and forge ahead.

Most of you know that I love good food, but I find that thinking about eating is even a challenge right now. I know how important staying rested and healthy is before starting the chemo treatments. I keep forcing myself to get up each day and either drink a nutritional shake with lots of berries, milk, banana, yogurt, and ground flax or have a bowl of oatmeal and a pear or orange, but it is not in me right now to rejoice in eating. It is part of my recovery plan. I try to reach for healthier things to eat during the day to help me recover more quickly. Mom, Jill, and I enjoyed a nice meal last evening of pork chops, rice, asparagus, and strawberry shortcake for dessert. Now that food finally tasted good!

It will be a bittersweet day for me tomorrow, celebrating Jill's fiftieth birthday and going for my first chemo meeting at 2:15 p.m. with Dr. Panwalkar. For those of you who missed it in yesterday's paper in the classified happy ads, we were successful in getting in a shout-out to Jill for her big five-oh! There was also an ad in our hometown Cando paper. I think Jill was surprised that I, along with a few other folks, could pull it off, considering the circumstances. A big "Thank you" to Arlene in

Cando and Shelley in Fargo for your great work and help in making the ads happen.

I am still at home today and tomorrow before my appointment and time will tell what my schedule of chemo sessions will be. I can honestly say that what lies ahead frightens me. If I were feeling better and sleeping better at night, I think my determination would be stronger. However, as many of you know, I am not a quitter. (Some would say I am like a dog with a bone.) So please know that I still intend to win this battle. It may knock me down a few times along the way, but I will cross the finish line the victor. I will try to keep you updated as this next phase progresses.

And speaking of finish lines, best of luck to everyone participating in the marathon this weekend. Last year's marathon was on my birthday, May 22, so I will just use the momentum from Saturday's event to carry me into a good day on Sunday celebrating my fifty-third birthday. Jill and I are usually on the corner of 8th Street and 13th Avenue. I will most likely be resting at home and praying for good weather and a great event for everyone involved. I also want to thank my family for being so supportive at this point in my life. They always have been there for me, but they are even more focused on getting me through this challenge now. I love you!

For all of you who have been by my side since I received this diagnosis, thank you for your continued prayers, good wishes, support, and compassion. They mean the world to me and my family. As I have said before, I am blessed to have you all in my life. Love you!

Sunday, May 22, 2011, 2:05 p.m., CDT

I Made It Another Year

When I was hearing and thinking about the predictions that the world may end on May 21, I had mixed feelings. I was bummed because my birthday was the day after the world was supposedly ending, and I was thinking that, on the other hand, I would not have to forge bravely ahead with my chemo and radiation if we all were gone.

So when I woke up this morning, I smiled a big smile and thought, "Good for you, Cindy Eggl. You (and the whole world) are here to celebrate your fifty-third birthday, and you can be brave and courageous and face down this diagnosis of breast cancer in the months ahead."

For those of you who remembered me with a phone call, e-mail, voice mail, card, or present for my birthday, thank you so much! No doubt each birthday I get to celebrate from this one on will be special, all part of the grateful feelings that are inherent to winning the battle of a lifetime. I appreciate your thoughtfulness.

On May 17, Jill celebrated her fiftieth birthday in style, and then she was gracious enough to share part of her special day going with Mom and me for my post-op appointment to see Dr. Panwalkar. At that appointment, the doctor confirmed my chemo and radiation treatments, a total of twenty weeks for chemo and five to six weeks for radiation. The first portion of chemo will be two types of chemo drugs administered two weeks apart for the first eight weeks and then a third chemo drug administered once a week for twelve weeks. The radiation treatments will follow the chemo treatments.

During my appointment, Dr. Panwalkar indicated that he wanted me to consider being part of a nationwide clinical trial, now in the third phase, for women with a HER-2/neu breast cancer marker of 1+ negative, of which I am one. If I am selected for the arm of the study of women with a 1+ negative marker, I will receive Herceptin, which, in the first two phases of the study, has shown promise for women who received this drug not having as great a chance of reoccurrence of breast cancer.

Additional blood tests, scans, and echocardiograms will be run on participants during the course of this trial, so I decided to sign on as a participant, following research and discussion of the pros and cons of participating. I have cleared the initial paperwork associated with the clinical trial, but I still must have a positive outcome from an echocardiogram and EKG test on Thursday, May 26, and blood tests on Thursday, June 2. Once I am cleared through those final tests, I should become a formal participant.

By choosing to be a participant, I will lengthen my course of treatment to a full year versus seven months, but if it means a lesser chance of my breast cancer returning and a way to help potentially improve chances for breast cancer patients with a 1+ negative HER-2/neu marker in the future, I am glad to be participating. I may be part of the arm of the trial that does not actually receive the Herceptin, but I would still receive all of the initial chemo and radiation treatments discussed with Dr. Panwalkar. Also, if at any time in the future things are not going well with the Herceptin administration, if I am chosen to participate in that arm, I can decide to end my participation in the clinical trial at any time.

I will go through a chemo orientation session on Friday, June 3, along with Mom and Jill, followed by another appointment with Dr. Panwalkar at 10:45 a.m. to firm up my treatment plan. My surgery to implant the port near my collarbone is scheduled for early Monday morning, June 6. The plan is to leave a needle in the port for use on Tuesday morning, June 7, during my first chemo session. This session will take six hours minimum on that day at the cancer center. From early explanations, the medical oncologist and chemo nurses make certain you are hydrated, if necessary, by an IV through the port. Then some anti-nausea medication is administered through the port, and finally, the chemo drug is given through the port.

Time will tell how well I tolerate the chemo treatments. I can only ask for your continued thoughts and prayers to help carry me through. I feel I am as mentally and physically strong as I can be at this time. As I have said in the past, now it is just walking the path from one procedure to the next.

I have tried to continue working at a pace that has kept me as healthy as possible, and I plan to attend the board meeting to take minutes on Monday, May 23, as well as work in the office as much as possible this next week.

Thank you, once again, to my family for their support and hours of caregiving and for the tremendous outpouring of your prayers, cards, e-mails, voice mails, remembrances, and compassion. So far, so good! I will continue to update you on my progress. Until then, take care. I love you!

Tuesday, May 31, 2011, 7:28 a.m., CDT

Good Things Come to Those Who Wait

I have been praying during this waiting and healing time that my mind, body, and spirit continue to grow in strength - I am resolved to endure what lies ahead. I still have moments when the pain at and around the surgical areas can take my breath away, and at other times, I feel like I could accomplish quite a lot, all within the parameters that my medical team has placed me under.

For instance, it was a complete joy, even though it was damp and on the cold side, when I rode with Jill to Rose Creek Golf Course and walked into the pro shop to greet the wonderful folks who work there. Matt, the PGA professional for the facility, handed me a key to a golf cart, and then I drove on the cart path watching and coaching while Jill golfed on Saturday and Sunday mornings. I was at peace knowing I could not golf for the time being, but I was also so happy just to be out on the course riding in a cart. I was diligent to keep the mosquitoes and cold away and to not get too carried away with telling Jill all the things I would fix. After all, she does have the much better swing and game of the two of us, so it is hard to find things to help her improve her game.

As I was driving the cart, I also wondered if we were going to be able to pull off the Cando Connection Golf Tournament, scheduled for Rose Creek Golf Course in Fargo, on June 18. We have a number of hole sponsors but not a lot of teams signed up right now, so I hope a number of additional people sign up in the next week or so to participate in our annual event. If you would like to register and play, I would sincerely appreciate your help. We can pair you together as teams if you don't have one already pulled together.

Hosting a successful event this year would be a major victory for me. As those of you who know me realize, it is all about the giveback for me and, in this case, the giveback to my hometown Cando area. I always joke with folks who tell me I am so positive that I cannot help be encouraging when I come from a place called Cando. Go to www.candoconnection.org to find the registration form under the 2011 Tournament tab. Even if you don't golf, you could join us for dinner at Rose Creek following the event. I would love to see you there!

I worked last week and intend to do the same this week. I believe it is hugely beneficial for me to stay in a forward-thinking, positive atmosphere, and my job and our missions provide an ideal place to accomplish that goal. I am blessed and grateful for all my job has brought to my life, especially now.

At times, it feels surreal, like I am living two separate lives, but then reality sets in, and I know that some rather challenging times lie ahead. I have prayed, planned, and organized as much as possible to try to not only help myself but those who have so lovingly surrounded me and will continue to be by my side as I go through each phase of this battle. Know that I have been trying to do everything within my power to stay as healthy, happy, calm, and determined as possible so that, when the time comes that I have to dig a little deeper, I can do so.

Your continued thoughts and prayers carry me from day to day. I am grateful. Thank you. Love you lots!

Friday, June 3, 2011, 4:05 p.m., CDT

Being Optimistic … Even When Plans Change

On Wednesday, June 1, I completed all of the required tests and blood work to be considered as a participant in the national clinical trial that Dr. Panwalkar suggested to me. A number of health factors are considered when enrolling a patient in one of these studies, and unfortunately, because of my recent blood pressure medication change and a concern about the timing of my previous PET scan, I was not chosen.

When I was notified of the decision, the same calm, peaceful feeling that has been with me since my diagnosis and has remained a constant for the past few weeks was solidly in place. I told the person calling me that I had placed this decision and all other medical procedures and tests in God's hands, and if it were his will that I not be a participant, than I was fine with that decision. I firmly believe that, if I were meant to participate, I would have been enrolled. Rest assured I will receive all of the chemo and radiation treatments that Dr. Panwalkar initially ordered to help me fight this battle, and I firmly believe that God will see fit to bless me with renewed health once I complete my journey.

This morning, Friday, June 3, 2011, Mom, Jill, and I participated in the chemo orientation session at the Roger Maris Cancer Center. Along with three men and their wives, Mom, Jill, and I were in the class, so the male patients made me feel a little outnumbered, but as usual, I held my own.

I smiled this morning as the educator during the orientation session referred me to the TLC American Cancer Society catalog because I was able to reassure her that I had the items I needed already in hand. I had started to cut my hair a little shorter, and I had embraced the fact that my appearance was going to change. In other words, I was my normal, organized self. It is nice to be in control of a few aspects of this journey. I received a large notebook with support materials to help guide us through the months ahead, just some light reading before I go to sleep each evening.

Another hurdle cropped up during my appointment with Dr. Panwalkar at 10:45 a.m. this morning. He told me my blood test from Wednesday indicated my liver function levels were a little out of range, and he questioned me about what medications I had been taking. When I reassured him I was not self-medicating and I was following his instructions, taking only my prescribed medications, over-the-counter drugs, and herbal green tea he had approved, he asked that I have a second blood test today to recheck the liver function and then changed several of my medications.

He took me off the pain medication oxycodone/Tylenol and ibuprofen and prescribed just oxycodone as my new pain medication. My follow-up blood test today indicated the liver function levels were still out of range, so Dr. Panwalkar ordered a recheck of my liver function through a blood test following the insertion of my port this coming Monday, June 6, at Sanford Same Day Surgery. I will be saying extra prayers that my liver function returns to normal and ask that, if you have some extra requests, you would also pray for a positive resolution to this new health concern for me as well.

I also came home with some cream to apply to my skin over the port area prior to my chemo sessions and two medications to help with fatigue and nausea afterwards. My first chemo session is scheduled for 9:00 a.m. this Tuesday, June 7. We have been told to plan to be at the cancer center for six hours for each of these four initial sessions. I have tried to embrace change in the past, not only in my professional life but also personally, and I am learning that I need to be resilient, strong, brave and adapt as health challenges arise.

I have had an opportunity to communicate with a number of good people in Cando, formerly from Cando, or who might have a Cando connection over the past few days. I was either trying to confirm their hole sponsorship, potentially secure a team of golfers, or even gather individual golfers we can pair with others for our golf tournament/dinner coming up on Saturday, June 18, 2011, at Rose Creek Golf Course in Fargo at noon. I can't begin to express my gratitude for the many positive comments and words of encouragement during each call. It is overwhelming to know what a tremendous team of supporters are thinking and praying for me during this time in my life. Thank you! If anyone is contemplating participating in our Cando Connection event, please consider making the decision to join us. We would love to have you golf and to see you.

I realize how blessed I have been with the many positive results and outcomes following my procedures and surgery so far. I know that, at the end of each day, when I lay my head down on my pillow, I should thank God for my overall health and pray he will carry me through what lies ahead.

As always, thank you for your continued thoughts, prayers, cards, e-mails, guestbook entries, and remembrances. I will continue to keep you informed as I move ahead in my journey. I love you!

Tuesday, June 7, 2011, 7:31 a.m., CDT

It Can Only Get Better from Here … I Hope!

I had a really rough day yesterday following the port implant surgery. I ended up in the emergency room yesterday afternoon, but a lot could not be done to help with the severe pain. I am not looking forward to chemo starting today because I am in so much pain. Hopefully, time will heal the areas that the port implant affected. All I can say is "Wow!" Maybe since I had so much trouble yesterday, the chemo side effects will be minimal today. I can only pray that will be the case.

I so hope I can get back to my more normal, positive self soon. Even I would not want to be around me yesterday afternoon and last night. Thank goodness for my big, blue recliner. It was a godsend, as were Jill, Mom, and Tom, my brother-in-law. Thank you for your continued thoughts and prayers. I love you!

CHEMOTHERAPY

Wednesday, June 8, 2011, 11:57 a.m., CDT

One Chemo Session Down … Fifteen to Go!

I slept well last night after a bout of nausea about 8:30 p.m. following my first day of chemo. I was able to reach the medical oncologist on call who was able to help guide me through the tough time with medication I already had in hand. So far, so good this morning. I am very tired, but I am trying to forge ahead on a few items, both work- and home-related, which keep me focused on positive things in my life. One day at a time and, sometimes, one hour at a time is how I tackle the fight right now.

I have to go for a shot at the cancer center this afternoon at 2:30 p.m. to help boost my white blood cell count. Thank you, Jamie, for agreeing to drive me, so Jill can be at work for meetings today and Mom gets a little rest as well.

My liver function has rebounded back 50 percent, which is good to know, so each bit of good news is a victory for me right now. I know I am early in the fight, so I am grateful that I feel as good as I do.

Thanks once again for all of your thoughts, prayers, and generosity in remembering me during this challenging time in my life. Either reading, writing to me, calling, or just plain listening to me talk mean the world to me because I know I am not in this battle on my own. No one can say that your love has not and will not surround me and carry me through during this time. I know I am blessed, and I am grateful. I love you!

Saturday, June 11, 2011, 6:37 a.m., CDT

What the Heck Just Happened?

On Friday morning, June 10, I rose with a fairly optimistic start with just a little bit of an appetite, drank a nutritional berry/banana shake, ate a bowl of instant cream of wheat, and decided to tackle the pieces of wallpaper that needed to be stuck down out in the hallway as I was making my morning walk back and forth for exercise. Thanks, Mom, for holding the various tools, paste, and so forth I needed to complete the task.

Once I finished that and sat down to work on the computer, things slowly went downhill from there. I was still feeling quite achy and not quite myself from the port placed on my right chest under the skin on Monday, June 6, my first chemo session on Tuesday, June 7, and a shot to boost my white blood cell counts on Wednesday, June 8. I have felt like I have a bad case of the flu. I have been battling nausea and fatigue, but I refuse to just lay around feeling sorry for myself. I intend to win this battle and be back to my normal self as soon as possible.

When the doctors put you on this much medication, it is important to know that you should continue to go to the bathroom as much as possible to clear your system. Suffice it to say, I learned through quite a bit of trial and error with what is on the market how best to deal with this element of my journey, and I will not let myself get to that point if I can ever help it again. I was miserable, and the thought of eating any type of food was beyond anything I have ever experienced, even when I have had a bad case of the stomach flu. Most of you know me. I love to eat. I just plainly love food, but yesterday was one of the worst days of my life when it came to having an appetite, not your normal (and I know that you are thinking "normal" is not part of who I am) Cindy at all.

I somehow slept through the night last night. Thank you, Mom, for your constant vigilance in making certain I was okay. The doctor's office had wanted me to go back to the emergency room if I did not feel better because it was thought I might have a bowel blockage, so I am grateful that did not occur in the middle of the night.

I am still somewhat in pain this morning, but I am trying to push through to do some work- and house-related things so I am not just lying around like a bump on a log. As I mentioned to my boss yesterday, it is amazing what all the medications do to your mind and system. But I refuse to just be sedentary and not be productive. I have been scared nearly to death about not getting infections and encountering lots of germs, so Mom has been wiping, cleaning, spraying, and trying to keep everything as sanitary as possible around the condo, and everywhere I go, I wipe down things and wash my hands incessantly. The only thing I have not had to do is wear a white gown with gloves, shoe covers, and so forth.

So for the time being, I have been working on some things from home for work and such. Hopefully, once I get past this first phase, I can be a little freer to be out and about. Thanks for your understanding and support, including thoughts, prayers, remembrances, and so forth. I appreciate it. Love you and miss you guys!

Tuesday, June 14, 2011, 7:22 a.m., CDT

Getting Ready for Round Two

I feel like today I might be back in the land of the living. I say that with a smile on my face. Even a few taste buds might be happy to try to work when I eat some food this evening. I realized I am factual with my journal entries because I am trying to help educate others who may be placed in this situation in the future, and sometimes, it might be more than you want to know. Bear with me because I am on numerous medications, and my way of sharing may not be what everyone would like to read or know about.

My ears do not always hear what the physicians and nurses are trying to say to me to try to help me, and even more frustrating is when I have a certain time frame in mind that I have heard when it was suggested I might start to feel better. And when I don't move along at that pace, I start to worry about other things that may be happening to me.

However, all in all, I count my blessings that I have you all on my team, thinking, praying, and supporting me, no matter what my journal entries or e-mails might say, and I hope at the end of the day you will forgive me if I have offended anyone in any manner.

I hope I may get permission to drive and take a short trip to the office tomorrow to check in, work a little, and just feel a little more normal before the weekend is upon us and we host the June 18 Cando Connection Golf Tournament at Rose Creek.

In other good news, I still have most of my hair left, and I can actually remember and carry on a conversation with someone and make sense during the course of the conversation. And depending on who I speak with, laughter may even occur. So I have come a long way over the past few days when, at times, I wasn't certain what was going on in my life.

My next lab draw is next Monday, June 20, and the next chemo session is Tuesday, June 21. It isn't a lot of time to recover and feel yourself, but I understand why and will try to be positive and brave as I was during the first session.

As always, I don't want one of you to think I do not sincerely appreciate and know in my heart all you have done for me to help me get this far in this journey. Your constant prayers, cards, calls, e-mails, guestbook entries, and remembrances have held me up as I have wandered in the dark some nights, wondering if the next six months will go any faster than this past week. I know I will make it, and I know you think and pray I will, too. I love you for everything. Thank you!

Monday, June 20, 2011, 7:50 a.m., CDT

What a Wonderful Day!

It was in the low eighties with barely a hint of wind and just a few white, puffy clouds in the sky. There were thirty-two players (eight teams) and twenty-one hole sponsors, and God saw fit to bless me with enough stamina, health, and, as I joked about (but was relieved), hair to make it through the Fourth Annual Impact-Cando Connection Fund Golf Tournament at Rose Creek this past Saturday, June 18. The three days leading up to the event, my energy level seemed to build little by little, and I believe that was because of the many prayers being offered up on my behalf. And to all those who took time to say prayers on my behalf, thank you so much. They truly carried me through the day.

Our Cando Connection event and giveback initiative have always meant a great deal to me, but even more so this year after getting my diagnosis and, at one time, debating whether it would be in my best interest to go forward with hosting the event. But am I ever glad that we did. I got the opportunity to thank the folks who so graciously shared their time, talent, and treasure to benefit the Cando area by participating in the event, and it also meant a lot to me to let people know how much I personally appreciated their kind words, thoughts, cards, remembrances, and prayers that have been and hopefully will continue to carry me through the tough times ahead.

A very dear person in my life orchestrated a special moment just prior to the start of the golf tournament. He asked that a sleeve of pink golf balls, each with a breast cancer awareness insignia, be distributed to each golfer in my honor. The thoughtfulness of that gesture deeply touched me, and it made me all the more grateful I have people like him in my life and by my side as I fight my way through this battle. Jill and I will update our website with photos from the golf event. You can find us at www.candoconnection.org. To those who made a donation to our Impact-Cando Connection Fund and in support of me making it through this year's event and my battle ahead, thank you so much!

I also want to thank Jennifer, my co-worker, for sharing a portion of her day to take photos at our event. They look great, Jennifer. We appreciate your continued support. And to Jill and Rusty, for being such great advisory board members to work with on this giveback endeavor, thank you for your patience and support. We did it!

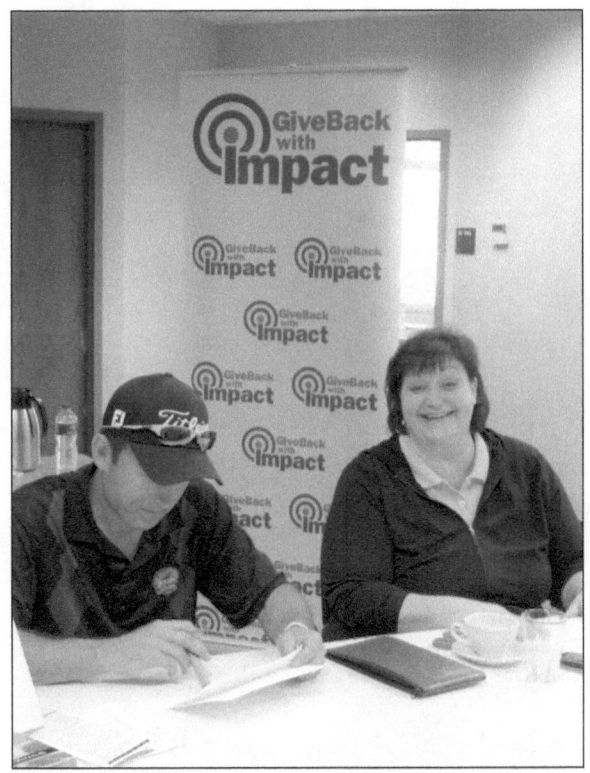

Rusty and Cindy at the registration table during the 2011 Impact-Cando Connection Golf Tournament.

In another instance, another dear friend came over to snap a photo of me for a sign and then walked in my honor during a recent Relay for Life event. She said my photo was near the starting line, and my luminary had the saying, "You Can-Do it" (pretty clever) written on it, along with my name. To Donna and her blisters and thoughtfulness, thank you so much. I have put up the photos she shared with me on my website.

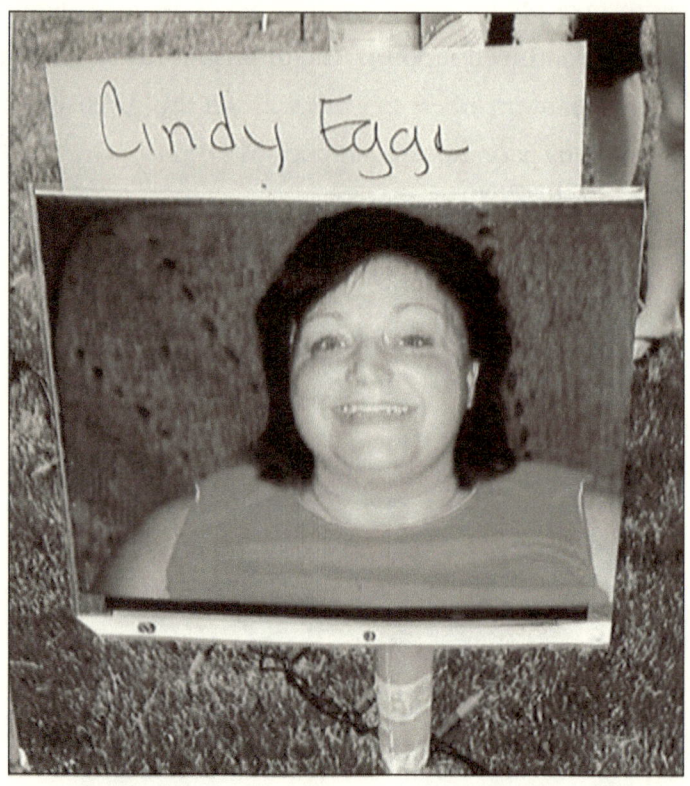

The sign placed by Donna, my neighbor, in my honor during the Relay for Life event held in 2011. What an incredibly thoughtful and generous way to honor someone going through a life-altering experience!

So, I go to the lab for a blood draw this morning to see how all the cells are doing and that everything else is in good shape for me to have my second chemo treatment tomorrow, Tuesday, June 21. Another dear friend, Lee, who has made certain I am entertained by either CDs, books, or music and have my mind taken off what I am going through during the six-hour process, has graciously donated an iPod.

Many others have reached out and thoughtfully remembered me with religious medals, prayer shawls, subscriptions, reading materials, funny stories, beautiful flowers and plants, food, gift certificates, guardian angels, good luck charms, pins, health tips, phone calls, e-mails, cards, guestbook entries, access to golf carts while at the course, and, most importantly, their continued prayers. Thank you for being such wonderfully compassionate and caring people. I am truly blessed by having you all in my life and on my side as I wake each day and pray it will be a good one. I know you are praying with me, and that gives me strength. I send my thanks, gratitude, and love to each of you for everything.

And finally to Mom, thanks for hanging in there with me, even when I am at my snarliest. (And yes, there have been a few of those moments.) I am glad God blessed me with you as my mom. I could not ask for a better one. I love you! I hope everyone has a great week. Love you!

Thursday, June 23, 2011, 11:07 a.m., CDT

Second Chemo Session Down ... Fourteen to Go!

All in all, things seemed to improve this time around in the second chemo process. I only had to have two sticks in my right arm for the blood draw on Monday to determine my overall cell counts. My veins like to go underground when they see the needle coming. On Tuesday, some of the anti-nausea medications (five different types) administered prior to my two types of chemo medications being given have been changed. I wore my "Chemo Sucks" button that my dear friend Shelley had given me in a pack of four designed specifically for this type of journey. Dr. Panwalkar and the nurses got a kick out of it.

I think Mom and Jill thought they had brought home the Energizer Bunny rather than Cindy Eggl following my chemo session because I was lit up and had trouble going to bed before 2:00 a.m. I even had Jill working on replacing lamps in some of our fixtures in the condo. (I have to use the right terminology because Jill is a lighting designer and she glares at me when I say bulbs instead of lamps.) I did some work for the office, and finally at 2:00 a.m., Mom looked at me and said, "Don't you think it is time for you to go to bed and get some rest," so I did, but I was back awake about 6:00 a.m. and still going strong.

That energy boost lasted until about 1:15 p.m. yesterday when I had to go back to the cancer center for my second Neulasta shot to help build my white blood cell count. I think that Mom, Jill, and I reminded each other that I was supposed to pick up my new medication at the cancer center pharmacy about eight times when I was there for my chemo session, but we all forgot to get it before we left. You are all just relieved to have gotten through the hours-long event, so we all walked out without it.

When Mom and I went back for my Neulasta shot yesterday, I remembered to wear another one of my new buttons that said, "I Love My Pain Meds," and that helped me remember to get my medication from the pharmacy. Amazing what small things can help you remember when you are in a fog.

Last night and this morning, I am dealing with headache, chills, and achy muscles and joints, but I am sticking to the medication schedule that Dr. Panwalkar has determined would work best. And I hope I will feel better much sooner than the last time. My taste buds are hanging in there better this time, but my hair is deciding it is time to head out or off, depending on how you want to think of it. I knew it was going to happen, so I am well prepared with my wigs, scarves, hats, and so forth so I will look more normal when it all falls out. If that is the worst of my worries, I will be doing well.

My liver function is back within normal range, but I will work to build up my hemoglobin by eating more red meat, raisins, or other natural foods and taking small doses of iron when I can tolerate taking it. All in all, Dr. Panwalkar said I am doing well for going through chemo so far, and I am grateful.

To all of you who continue to read, reply, call, write, or remember me in various ways, thank you, but most especially, thank you for your prayers. I know from his emails that Jim is saying his prayer for me on 25th Street on the way to work each day – I am grateful! That is it for now. Just know I love you all lots!

Friday, July 1, 2011 6:01 a.m., CDT

I Better Get Going While the Going Is Good!

My next lab draw is today, Friday, July 1, and my next appointment and chemo session is scheduled for Tuesday, July 5. Jill and I plan to enjoy the weekend in Fargo, and we will pick up Mom in Grand Forks on either July 3 or 4 so she is back with me for the next round of chemo.

For the past week, I have felt pretty good, and I decided the saying, "I better get going while the going is good," really applies at this point in my life. I find that, although this diagnosis and the manner in which you are medically treated profoundly changes your perspective on things and how you look at your life, the core of your being remains the same. If you were a workaholic before the diagnosis, you most likely will continue to be one during and after the diagnosis. There just seems to be an urgency to get things done more quickly. As I have alluded to earlier, patience has never really been a strong suit of mine, but I truly have improved in that area (or at least I think I have). But my desire to continue to do things with excellence, focused dedication and a passion for the project I am doing at the moment has not changed.

So, over the past few days, Jill and I tackled a few items in our condo, but mostly Jill, mind you. I have been cheering her on from the sidelines, holding the flashlight, and handing her the screwdriver, wrench, nut, washer, screw, chain, or whatever happens to be in the box of goodies that we are working on at the moment. We installed a new fan motor in my bathroom, a new overhead fan and light fixture in her bedroom, a new door closing mechanism on our screen door, and we moved our sound system to a different configuration. We also completed the updates on the www.candoconnection.org website with the 2011 tournament information following our event and prepared a full-page press release for the local newspaper, which should run this weekend over the Fourth of July. We spoke with recipients of the grant designations from our tournament held June 18 for the Impact-Cando Connection Fund. I should also mention that I have been in the office working nearly full time. "I better get going while the going is good" has worked in my favor. It has kept me focused and looking forward to better, more normal days ahead, and I am grateful to be busy and feeling as good as I am.

Jill and I joined two of our cousins and their wives—Jim and Sue who live in Fargo and Jack and Diane who live in California—for dinner this past Wednesday. Diane just completed her battle with ovarian cancer in April of this year, and she has been a wealth of knowledge when it comes to dealing with the chemo aspect of my diagnosis. She told me in a recent phone call that they would be traveling to North Dakota (Cando) to be with family for my Aunt Eileen's birthday celebration over the Fourth of July. She also said they would come to Fargo so we could have dinner and be together to share notes on our battles with cancer. Even cooler, Sue is also a breast cancer survivor of nearly twenty years, so if that weren't an inspirational evening for me, I don't know what would be. We all had a wonderful time, and I am grateful they made the trip so we could be together.

A number of other people have survived and thrived following their fight with cancer, and they have reached out by e-mail, a card, a phone call, or in person to share their stories. And each and every one has been an inspiration to me. Your courage, wisdom, encouraging words, and prayers have lifted me up at times when I might have been feeling vulnerable or even times when I was feeling good. And it reaffirmed what my future holds as well. Thank you. You all know who you are, and I respect and admire your tenacity, strong will to beat this disease, and willingness to reach out to others who fight a similar battle.

So I prepare for the third chemo session and ask for your continued thoughts and prayers as I tick one more off the list and strive for the finish line. I pray that all of you have a healthy and safe Fourth of July holiday weekend. Thank you for all you have done to bring me this far. Take care. I love you!

Saturday, July 9, 2011, 5:17 a.m., CDT

Chemo Session Three Is Done

For those of you who have been following me in my journey with my breast cancer battle, you know that, when I was first diagnosed, I was told I would be going through a series of sixteen chemo sessions. Part of each treatment is receiving a Neulasta shot just twenty-four hours after each chemo session for the first four treatments to help boost the white blood cell count and make it possible for me to continue my treatments. The Neulasta shot has been the most challenging part of my treatments so far, with flu-like symptoms for two to five days, depending on how the rest of me feels. After the first session, it was about five days. After the second and third sessions, it was about two to three days. And hopefully for my fourth session, now scheduled for July 19 with the Neulasta shot on July 20, it will be a shorter version of time I am affected. Time will tell. Additionally, Dr. Panwalkar told me that because I am having my last twelve chemo sessions on a weekly basis, if my white blood cells hang in there, I most likely won't have to have the Neulasta shots. I will say extra prayers for the strength of my white blood cells.

A number of people have asked about the process and drugs currently being administered prior and during my chemo sessions. I generally have labs drawn either the day before or several days before if there is a holiday or scheduling conflict. Then I meet with Dr. Panwalkar the morning of my scheduled chemo, and he confirms if I am able to go through the next round of chemo that day.

So an hour before I head out the door with my family members in tow (bless their souls for being there with me through this ordeal), the first drug I apply is a layer of Lidocaine cream on the skin over my port. The port was implanted under the skin on my chest near my collarbone to help save my arm and other veins from going through the rigors of chemo drugs, which can burn skin and tissue if your veins do not hold up. The port has worked extremely well, and it is now causing only minimum issues such as neck spasms or being a little sore after chemo. I handle that with a half dose of Diazepam (or Valium) as a muscle relaxer when needed and a two hundred-milligram dose of ibuprofen. When the going gets really tough, it is back to a half dose of the Oxycodone, but I rarely need to take that at this point in time.

So when I get into the chemo room, the nurse counts to three and inserts the butterfly needle into the port area. (And I can honestly say very little pain has been associated with that process. Thank God for the Lidocaine.) Then we start the process with what I call the "ramp-up" drugs prior to the chemo drugs being administered.

The ramp-up drugs include Dexamethasone (a steroid drug) to primarily help prevent nausea, increase appetite, reduce swelling and inflammation, and help prevent or treat allergic reactions to certain drugs. The next ramp-up drug, Palonosetron, is also an anti-nausea medicine. And the final two drugs administered through the port prior to the chemo drugs are Zantac and Benedryl. By the time I get those and they start to work, I am pretty much out of the picture, laying back in my reclining chair and just getting ready for the drugs to be administered, or, as Mom or Jill would attest, sleeping my way through the next part of the session.

The first chemo drug being used for my breast cancer, Doxorubicin, looks like a red-dyed chemo drug. The nurse covers herself from head to toe in protective layers and safety glasses while I lay there in my street clothes hoping all goes well. (It's a little scary but a necessary evil.) Two vials of that good stuff go in the line. This drug is part of a group of chemo drugs known as anthracycline antibiotics, which slows or stops the growth of cancer cells.

Then it is on to the Cyclophosphamide, which is mixed in and administered through an intravenous bag. It is an alkylating agent drug to help stop cancer cells from growing, causing them to die. I count on those last two drugs to get me back on my feet and onto better health in the future.

So as I come out of my stupor following all the drugs, I generally leave about five to six hours after we arrive at the Roger Maris Cancer Center, feeling a little bit wobbly but walking on my own and being grateful for making it through another session.

Dr. Panwalkar has also prescribed several drugs that I use at home following my chemo treatments and after the Neulasta shots. I take Dexamethasone for up to three days after the chemo session, and I take Prochlorperazine Maleate only as needed for nausea. I am grateful for both of those drugs. They truly have made a difference in how I have been able to cope following each chemo session so far.

I promise the next time I see any of you that I won't quiz you on the drugs, but a number of people had asked about what happens during the course of chemo, and what drugs were being administered, so I wanted to be able to answer your questions.

I don't know what the treatment drug or associated drugs will be during the upcoming twelve-week chemo session where I go once a week. I am certain more good drugs are in my future, and I will share that information when I get my hands on it, so to speak.

Other than the very detailed information above, I have been doing as well as can be expected. A few blood tests are either above or below the normal range. Hemoglobin is down to 9.8, which is to be expected because the bone marrow is not functioning as it normally would be. Potassium level is just slightly down, but bananas and I will become much better friends for the time being. And my glucose level is quite high (180) due to the extra steroid drugs. Dr. Panwalkar has asked me to do a fasting lab draw the next time around to see where my levels are at on Friday, July 15, and I am certain he will make corrections or add some drug if needed to address any issues if they remain out of range.

So three chemo sessions down and thirteen to go. A step at a time, recovery in between, some really fun wigs, taste buds that are kind of hanging in there with me, some good energy levels most of the time, and a hugely positive attitude. I know I will get through this.

As I always request at the end of these journal updates, I ask for your continued thoughts and prayers that things may continue to go as well as possible, and I will be stronger and better after this battle for having gone through it. Some of you may have heard me sing "Wind Beneath My Wings" some time in your life, and you all have certainly been that for me, and I am eternally grateful. I love you all very much!

Wednesday, July 20, 2011, 5:30 p.m., CDT

Chemo Session Four Done ... Phase I Complete!

I have now completed the fourth double chemo session and phase one of my breast cancer battle. Yippee! Something wonderful to celebrate!

My chemo session was yesterday, July 19. Vicki, my older sister, checked in on Monday morning to make certain I was doing okay, and I told her, if I were not calling her, that no news was good news. I have also imparted the same sentiment to my brothers Scott and Mark, Mark's wife Carla, their family, Aunts Judy and Nita, and their families. If I am not calling you, think only good things.

My mom decided to stay in Cando to keep the motel, which has had really wonderful business over the last few weeks, running smoothly at her eighty years of age and after fifty-one years of business, and to give herself a chance to catch up on a number of things, including giving her knees a rest as best she can. She has to walk a long set of stairs to get up to our condo when she is with us, and it is hard for her, so a little time back home just to regain her footing in a number of ways was in order.

Jill accompanied me to my chemo session yesterday morning and early afternoon, and I went on my own today for my fourth and, hopefully last, Neulasta shot. It all depends on how my white blood cell count hangs in there through the next phase of chemo if another one of these shots has to be administered.

There will be no break in between the first and second phases of chemo. I start the twelve-week, once-per-week sessions on August 2, and I will hopefully complete phase two on October 18 if all goes well. I keep telling myself not to get too far ahead of myself, but I am staying positive and focused on the future, being the consummate planner and organizer that I am known to be.

I do have some chicken down still left on my head, as well as some eyebrows and eyelashes, so I am glad to know that not everything has gone "by the by" (one of my favorite sayings). Jill and I joked that I may have to have Lacey, my hairstylist, trim my hair if it gets too long.

We also have not had any grass growing under our feet. This past Saturday, we laid laminate hardwood flooring in our kitchen with just the two of us, with an assist by Amanda and John, who loaned us their triangle and square, which came in very handy to make certain things were squared up. On Sunday, we laid the same flooring in the foyer of our condo. I do want everyone to know that we invested in the best kneepads that money could buy for Jill because, with my port for chemo being implanted, I could not be on my knees or with my head down for long periods of time. So kudos to Jill for carrying the heavy load on this home improvement project. It looks wonderful, and we are very proud that we could accomplish it on our own. Who says two women in their fifties can't do home improvement projects?

So as I always sign off in these journal and e-mail entries, I am grateful and blessed to be doing so well through my chemo treatments. If my blood work hangs in there and the next series of chemo sessions go well, I will be thrilled. I was told at the cancer center today that I was doing extremely well. Evidently, some patients who go through this don't know their names, what day it is, where they are from, and so forth, so I feel doubly blessed and know that all of your thoughts and prayers are paying off. Thank you for keeping me on your prayer lists and generally in your prayers. I appreciate it so much.

Here is hoping that you are staying as cool as possible in this hot weather. I love all of you very much for all you have done for me.

Tuesday, July 26, 2011, 7:00 a.m., CDT

A Little Wake-up Call

After talking with my oncologist's office yesterday, my medication was slightly adjusted, and I was asked to go to the lab this morning to have my hemoglobin reading checked. The last two nights have been a little rough in terms of dealing with nausea, fatigue, headache, chills, and so forth, and my taste buds have abandoned me once again, so everything tastes like it is hot or cold and not much else. Not too much fun eating right now. But like a few other things, it's a necessary evil, so I am choosing to continue to eat more fruits and vegetables and my favorite go-to food item, bread. It's probably not the best thing in the world, but it is most satisfying for my system at the moment. Oh, the little things in life that make me feel better!

Now, my bone marrow is not producing red blood cells anywhere close to where they would normally be, so if my hemoglobin blood work comes in this morning below 8.5, I will need blood transfusions to get me back on my feet with more energy. This development is not totally unexpected, but I am feeling just a bit more vulnerable than I have been feeling. I don't know if I should pray for the blood transfusions or not. If they will make me feel better and less fatigued, perhaps that is what I should focus my prayers on. Either way, I am trying to maintain my positive attitude, but just when you think that things are going along swimmingly, God shakes you up and reminds you that you are in a breast cancer battle.

I was really bummed out yesterday when I had to call my friend Phil and tell him that I couldn't participate in his camp for kids this year because I couldn't be out in the sun for periods of time and my energy level was quite low. I have so enjoyed being part of the team that timed the forty-yard dash for the past three years at his camp, so that was a tough call for me to make yesterday. I hope to be back next year with my forty-yard dash partner, Mark, once I get past this battle.

My next lab after today is next Monday, August 1, and the first of twelve weekly chemo sessions is Tuesday, August 2, with the third (new) type of chemo coming into play. Just know I appreciate your continuing thoughts and prayers, and I am grateful for everything everyone has done so far to help me get to this point. Have a great rest of the week. I love you!

Wednesday, July 27, 2011, 6:15 a.m., CDT

Just Wanted You to Know

I don't normally journal more than once a week, but the outpouring of e-mails, calls, and personal visits yesterday prompted me to send a quick update to let you know that my hemoglobin reading came back at 9.3, well above the 8.5 or below reading that would have required blood transfusions, so I did not have to go in. Whatever prayers you said were obviously the right ones. As I mentioned yesterday in my journal and e-mail update, I wasn't certain what to pray for, but obviously my prayers were answered. After Dr. Panwalkar and Andrea, his nurse, slightly adjusted my medication yesterday morning, I started feeling improved yesterday afternoon and slept much better last night as well. I am grateful and feel blessed.

I think I have a guardian angel over at the lab by the name of Mary. She told the other lab technician yesterday that he could register me for the lab draw but said I was her patient and she would be doing the blood draw. We had a wonderful conversation yesterday that put me at ease, and she reassured me that I would have my results back as soon as possible so I didn't need to worry longer than necessary about the blood transfusions. This same person gave me a hug when I left after my last blood draw two weeks ago. Sometimes God just puts the right people in your life at the right time, and I have had more than my fair share of those people crop up in the last few months since I was diagnosed. Maybe I was just not as aware of the kind and compassionate folks I encountered every day. I guess that is another good thing that has come from going through this breast cancer fight.

My oncologist's office has told me to back off on expending my energy for this week and weekend leading into the start of my next series of chemo sessions. So any home improvement projects, cleaning, and so forth will be on the back burner for the time being (heavy sigh), which includes staying here in Fargo this weekend rather than heading to Cando, which I was hoping to do. They told me my health was to come first, and believe it or not, I do listen to what my doctor and his nurse have been telling me.

For all of you who contacted me and prayed for me, especially over the last few days, thank you! I sincerely appreciate your words of encouragement and prayers, and they hopefully will continue as I forge ahead with my battle. Take care. Love you!

Wednesday, August 3, 2011, 6:15 a.m., CDT

Next Chemotherapy Series Underway (Fifth Chemo Done)

And I am off and running on the second series of chemo drug treatments. (For those of you counting along with me, this was the fifth of the total of sixteen I am scheduled to go through.) Once again on Monday morning, Mary greeted me with a big smile when I registered and then had to make only one attempt for the blood draw from my hand, which meant we were off to a great start on this second series of chemo treatments. Just a tiny little indication there was anything drawn and no black-and-blue mark. Progress in the right direction!

Lab test results came back, and everything was looking pretty good, including my hemoglobin, which went up from 9.3 to 9.4. (It must be the iron and all the red meat I have been eating.) Dr. Panwalkar told me that number could vary by several tenths of a point from blood draw to blood draw. In my mind, it was a positive thing, so I am going with my gut feeling and just feeling grateful. All other numbers looked fine, including an additional thyroid test to make certain my nonfunctioning thyroid was still in range through all of this, and it was. Yeah! White blood cell count was good, too.

So, Mom, Jill, and I met with Dr. Panwalkar yesterday (Tuesday, August 2) morning, we reviewed the schedule for the next twelve weekly chemo treatments and the drug that will be administered along with the other ramp-up and follow-up drugs. Jill was relieved to hear I would not be taking Dexamethasone in large doses because it generally gives me extra energy and she has been working hard to keep up. She's kind of kidding about that. She has carried the heavy load through all of this. But she did jokingly ask Dr. Panwalkar if she could get something similar so she could survive my treatment schedule, too, if I were staying on that drug. We all laughed about that request.

For this new chemo treatment, I will only need a blood draw every three weeks, and I will see Dr. Panwalkar every three weeks for monitoring. The weeks in between, I will go for the chemo treatment only and will get Paclitaxel, which is thought to work by interfering with microtubules, part of the internal scaffolding that cells need when they divide into two cells. Over time, this leads to cell death. Because cancer cells divide more quickly than normal cells, this drug more likely affects them more than normal cells.

I was given about five ramp-up drugs yesterday, very similar to those administered during the first four chemo treatments, and I was infused the new drug at a slower rate to watch for any allergic reactions I might have. The oncology nurse, Sister Julie, Mom, Jill, and I all prayed over the cancer drug before it was administered yesterday, and those prayers must have been answered because I came through the treatment just fine. I had a bit of a headache right afterwards, but Dr. Panwalkar told me to try taking two Advil (two hundred milligrams) rather than one, and that got rid of the headache. Other than that, I had great energy last night, following a short nap yesterday afternoon, and feel quite good yet this morning,

Side effects of this drug may include:

- Nausea (which I already have a drug at the ready to help combat that effect)

- Potential sores in the mouth or on the lips

- Some intestinal issues (where dehydration is a concern)

- Nerve damage potentially of the hands or feet

- Hand-foot syndrome (including peeling, blistering, or sores on the skin)

- Heart rhythm issues

- Lower red blood cell and platelet counts

I will monitor all of these things closely, and I have been asked to stay in contact with my doctor and phone the nurse if symptoms start to appear. They also said I might have days that I would be achier, which Advil would help control, or feel fatigued, which rest would help cure.

Now that I have provided a synopsis of the new drug being administered, please know that, all in all, I have been doing well. I have been working full time at my job. We are just finishing up with some installation work in our kitchen. (Jill and I finally had to call in the professionals.) And our great-nephew and great-niece are staying with Vicki and Tom (my sister and brother-in-law, their grandparents) for two weeks, so lots of very positive things are going on in my life right now. I have also had a chance to see my two nieces, Lissa, who dropped off her children for their stay in Fargo, and Betsy, who was home several weeks ago and accompanied me for one of my Neulasta shots at the cancer center and will be back in Fargo for a few days starting Wednesday evening. I have made it a point to regularly talk with all of my family members and reassure them, if they don't hear from me that is good news.

The same holds true for all of you who have so thoughtfully but compassionately followed my progress. I cannot imagine going through this process without all of you—my family; boss; coworkers; board, committee, and members at work; friends; former coworkers; business acquaintances; classmates; Cando Connections; and the many people who have crossed my path, through the grace of God, along the way. You all have helped carry me through and have enriched my life by being in it and with your thoughts, prayers, and encouragement.

I felt blessed to be able to visit with my cousin and classmate, Erin, from Valley City yesterday, who graciously offered to come and visit following my chemo treatment. We had a wonderful time, and that visit hammered home the importance of staying in touch with the people God has seen fit to place in your life, no matter at which stage of your life. You just never know what tomorrow will bring, so my best advice is to not fritter it away. Grasp the opportunities to interact. You never know how what you say or do—a hug, a prayer, an e-mail, a note, a card, or, quite simply, just being in a person's presence—may affect someone.

As I always sign off, I sincerely appreciate everything everyone has done to bring me this far in this battle. I go to bed each night and wake each morning knowing how blessed I am, and I have God and all of you to thank for that feeling and my progress toward victory. Thank you! Love you!

Wednesday, August 10, 2011, 6:03 a.m., CDT

And Then There Were Ten

Ten chemotherapy treatments left! I made it through my sixth one, the second of twelve of the new type, yesterday. All in all, things went well. I did encounter a bit of an issue about halfway through the procedure with some chest heaviness and pain down my left arm. The nurse suspended my treatment until she spoke with Dr. Panwalkar, who ordered an EKG and blood test to check my enzyme level for potential heart muscle damage, a potential side effect of this chemo drug. The very good news is that the EKG came back as normal, and the blood enzyme test was within range, so all is well at this time. It was a little scary, but we (the rest of my cancer fighting team and me) always err on the side of caution. That is a huge comfort when you are sitting in the chair and you don't know what is happening at the time and following the treatment.

I continue to be able to work full time. (It isn't because I am being forced to. My boss, Pat, and all of the rest of the folks associated with what I do at work could not be more supportive, and I am thankful.) It continues to give me a positive, forward-looking peace of mind that is helping to carry me through my journey. I am grateful I have my job and our missions are so positive and uplifting. God truly smiled on me when I was chosen to become part of my work team.

I have had news this week from other folks in my life that will be fighting cancer battles of another nature, and I ask that you keep us all in your prayers. You just never know when you may get this type of news. It is always unsettling. The most important thing you can do is to reach out to others to ask for their prayers, stay as positive and looking forward to the future as possible, and then fight with everything you have within you to win the battle.

I continue to hear from many of you through e-mail, guestbook entries, cards, phone calls, and thoughtful gifts. Such as the box I received from my former co-worker, Mary, a talented woman who shaped the letters "HOPE" out of various natural resources on her latest vacation, photographed them, placed those photos into a four-picture frame, and mailed it off to me with a lovely card. It came to me out of the blue, at just the right time, to inspire me to get through a fairly rough Thursday through Sunday last week. This chemo works in a different way where I am much more fatigued with the trade-off of not having to have a Neulasta shot and not feeling as nauseated. So I choose to find the silver lining in this cloud, and I am resting more on the weekends so I have the energy to continue to work. Some would say I am doing this my own wrong way, but I know it is right for me, and that is important right now.

"All in good time" is my latest favorite phrase, which, when I translate, means I will make it through my battle and hopefully will be back to the normal me by the end of the year, minus most of my hair but still smiling, positive, focused, and a better person for having gone through what I just did.

For those of you who have shared your own cancer battle stories with me and to those of you who have helped your loved one through this situation, I once again want to say thank you. You inspire, reach down, and pull us up to a more positive train of thought, such an important component in our cancer battle. Continue to share your stories. There are a lot more of us out there than you know who are listening to you and need that extra bit of encouragement.

I feel your prayers, I am grateful for your thoughts, and I will continue to fight with all that I am to get through this battle. Thanks for being there for me. I appreciate it more than you know. Love you!

Tuesday, August 16, 2011, 9:25 p.m., CDT

One-Fourth through Second Chemo Series

Jill said to me the other day that she thought time was going by fairly quickly and she hoped I felt that way too in regard to my chemo treatments. I did look at her rather incredulously and said, "Really?" She said it seemed like the weeks were just flying by, which is generally how you feel about the summer months in North Dakota. I said that, all in all, time had gone by fairly quickly, except on the days I am achy, have chemo, feel very fatigued, and have swollen or painful bones, muscles and joints, and some nausea. However, I have very little to complain about in regard to how this process has unfolded. I am, after all, one-fourth of the way through the second chemo series with just nine chemo sessions left. October 18, here I come!

I have had several areas of concern crop up over the last several days, including a very painful spot on my lower right breast and under my right arm (the opposite side of where my breast cancer was initially diagnosed), but I hope it is chemo-related with it just doing its job. And, I have had a few stitches pop up from my port incision, and one of my oncology nurses wants to make certain that it is still functioning well, which will be checked next Tuesday morning (August 23) at 7:00 a.m., just prior to my next appointment with Dr. Panwalkar at 8:15 a.m.

Trust me, if there are any issues, we will all get to the root of them and work to make corrections. No stone left unturned in this saga! And then it is on to my ninth chemo session at 9:15 a.m. next Tuesday as well.

I feel fairly good yet this evening and hope to complete my workweek in the office through Friday. I have been working full time, a positive place to go in the morning and be in during the day, and you just never know when you might get thrown another curveball, so I am persisting in doing my job while I feel well enough to be there and work.

We are also dealing with a major sewer separation project that will disrupt potential water to our condo building and travel routes with only one driveway open behind our building to the north and no street access in front of our building, not to mention the fact that South University, our main driving route, is also under major road construction all for the next month. I think the saying, "When it rains, it pours," is appropriate about now. Come to think of it, that saying would be true for our whole summer so far. We have been in contact with the City of Fargo, and we hope to reduce some potential safety concerns in utilizing our driveway as the main source of leaving and returning to our condos, as well as confirming the water source for us on the days our access is restricted or is completely shut down will be adequate and safe. One less thing I needed to worry about during this time in my life, but hopefully it won't be as bad because we planned well in the beginning. Time will tell!

Almost daily, I receive cards, e-mails, phone calls, and personal well-wishes. It is uplifting to know how many people are pulling for me and humbling to know that they are thinking and praying for me through my journey. I don't know about all of you, but it seems like December is a long way away to complete all of my medical procedures. My patience has been tested in more ways than I can possibly count, but that is one of the things that is most important to have about now. So, I put a smile on my face, look forward to the next step, and just thank God that I have him and all of you in my life beside me.

My most sincere thanks to everyone, most especially, Jill, who has been and will be by my side getting me through each appointment. And I know that, if I need to reach out and ask, I can count on the rest of my family, friends, coworkers, and many others who would gladly offer to help when needed. It's quite a comfort when I go to sleep at night and wake up in the morning. I am so very grateful and send my thanks and appreciation to you all. Love you!

Tuesday, August 23, 2011, 8:32 p.m., CDT

Another Milestone Reached

Today's chemo session was my eighth out of sixteen treatments, so I am halfway through my chemo journey. All I can say is, "Yahoo!"

I started my day with a 7:30 a.m. appointment with interventional radiology, which checked the port implanted on my upper right chest and confirmed it was still in place and functioning as expected. They then proceeded to pull through and clip off a number of stitches that had popped up through my incision. It's not so bad and a relief to know that I didn't have to undergo another procedure to reposition the port.

I proceeded to my 8:15 a.m. appointment with Dr. Panwalkar with Jill in tow. I had a visit from my phone nurse, Andrea, who has seen me through a number of worrisome side effects of the chemo drugs. She and I have a wonderful relationship, and we laugh quite a bit, even when I am scared witless about the effects the chemo drugs are having on my body. She's a nice woman doing a tough job very well!

Dr. Panwalkar joined us and imparted that all of my blood work and numbers were looking good. I guess I had eaten enough beef and iron to raise my hemoglobin back up to 9.7 from 9.3, where it was based on my last blood test three weeks ago. Another thing to celebrate! Then Dr. Panwalkar told me he was taking me off one of my favorite ramp-up drugs, Dexamethasone. It helped prevent allergic reactions to the chemo drug, acted as an anti-nausea medication, and gave me extra energy to carry me through Tuesday and Wednesday of each week. He did leave me on one other lower-dose steroid to help with anti-nausea and allergy reactions so I didn't get left on an island, stranded and alone. Thanks, Dr. Panwalkar!

I made it through my eighth chemo session and proceeded home to rest for a few hours this afternoon. I don't have the extra energy I normally would have, but all in all, it feels pretty good. Dr. Panwalkar did talk about the cumulative effects of my chemotherapy drugs and that they would continue to build in my system, which will result in me feeling more fatigued as I continue down this path. I am also losing more hair from my fuzzy head and a few more brow and eyelashes. However, this was all part of what I knew was coming down the line, so I have been prepared. Just as a reminder, Jill has offered to help me pencil on my eyebrows, but for those of you who saw my demonstration of what she was threatening to do, unless she comes into my room in the middle of the night, she will not get close to my eyebrows anytime soon. I guess I will do as well as I can to look somewhat normal on my own.

God has a way of adding a little more drama to my life periodically so I am not totally focused on my own journey. I have lost sleep worrying and praying for positive resolutions to each of these situations:

- My mom went for a follow-up eye appointment and was not able to see the big "E" on the eye chart with her left eye, so she had to continue her eye injections for wet macular degeneration. Tonight, she looks like she was in a fight with her eye very bloodshot and black and blue on the skin just to the left of her eye. In good news, she has already regained some of her central vision as of tonight. Fight on, Mom!

- My brother and sister-in-law, Mark and Carla, who live in South Carolina and own property on Fripp Island, a barrier island just south of Charleston, South Carolina, are hoping not to be profoundly impacted by Hurricane Irene, and as of tonight, the models seem to show a more northerly impact closer to North Carolina. The extra prayers are paying off for them. And just for information sake, Mark and Carla promised not to ride out the storm, which I was grateful to hear. Thank you!

I still have my moments when I stop and think about what I am going through, and it almost seems surreal. Then I get an e-mail from a co-worker who uses these sentences. (Please note the strong encouragement, and she used pink lettering in recognition of a breast cancer battle):

Your number-one focus right now is getting yourself healthy and feeling better. We all know you're doing your best and trying to ignore the fatigue and soreness when you're in the office, but rest does amazing things for our bodies. Keep your chin up, your eyes looking forward, and your feet planted firmly on the ground. You'll get through this. You know you will. You have to. There is no choice. Tomorrow is a new day, and this too shall pass!

After reading that, I cannot help but win this battle, which you all know has been my number-one goal all along. With your continued support and prayers, I will win. You can count on me to stay strong, mentally, physically, and spiritually. I am profoundly grateful; not only for my coworkers' support, but for all of the support I have received.

Thank you for continuing to reach out to others and me, saying your prayers, and doing all the extra things you do to encourage others and me as well. Today was another good day with another huge milestone reached, and I could not be more proud to have you on my team and by my side. Here is to eight more weeks flying by and cheering for a successful completion of chemotherapy on October 18. Love you!

Friday, August 26, 2011, 6:30 a.m., CDT

A Hurdle to Jump

Just as things seemed to be going along smoothly, a hurdle was thrown up for me to get over. On Wednesday, the day after my chemo session, my lips and tongue started to get numb, like I had been injected with Novocain. By 4:30 p.m., I called Dr. Panwalkar's office, only to be told they felt it was nerve damage, a side effect of my latest chemo drug. I was prescribed a new drug, which also had some concerning side effects, to try to counteract the nerve damage. In addition, I was asked to go through a brain MRI yesterday (Thursday) to make certain no other complication was occurring. Thankfully, that scan came back as normal. I have been told that, because I am only fifty-three, there is a good chance I will recover the feeling in my lips and tongue. As a vocalist and someone who does interact verbally with others as part of my job and as a volunteer on other projects, I hope I will fully recover. I hope adjustments will be made to the chemo drug so I don't have further nerve damage in my hands and feet, where most patients have trouble. Leave it to me to be different yet again!

My mom is also having trouble with her left eye and continual bleeding. She will see a specialist this morning to see what our next steps should be to stop the bleeding and try to restore the vision more completely in that eye.

Thank you for your continued prayers. Mom and I plan to hang in there, being brave and good patients, all in the hopes of good outcomes. Thanks for being by our sides. We appreciate it. Love you!

Wednesday, August 31, 2011, 6:35 a.m., CDT

I Wonder Why?

Many times in the last five months, I have wondered. "Why?" At times, my journey has seemed surreal. It is as if I am watching myself go through each test, procedure, surgery, and chemo treatment from a distance, participating because I have no choice if I intend to survive this breast cancer diagnosis.

I have wondered why God chose me to walk this path. I wondered why both Dr. Bouton and Dr. Panwalkar told me that the breast cancer had been growing for between two to four years and I was fortunate enough that it had spread to only one lymph node and not throughout my body. I wondered why after doing all the right things to try to prevent this disease through mammograms, annual exams, and monthly self-breast exams that no one, including me, had caught my cancer earlier.

Then after pondering for these many months, I resigned myself to the fact that God did choose me for a reason, perhaps to continue to educate people I meet as I live my surreal life. Or perhaps I will serve as an example to others that they too can endure the rigors of the diagnosis—tests, surgery, chemo treatments, and radiation—and still continue to live their life, only to become a better person for having gone through it. Trust me, I have had much to think about, and the answers have not all been clarified yet. Time, no doubt, will provide that clarification.

On a brighter note, I was delighted when my niece Betsy showed up at my door to take me for my chemo treatment yesterday. She had driven in the evening before from the Twin Cities and offered to help when Jill could not get away from work to take me for my session. I could have called several family members who had offered to take me, but Betsy got to see the full treatment yesterday and was a trooper. Thanks, Beez!

I also had a wonderful visit during my treatment from two of my former coworkers, Mary and Jane, from Sanford Foundation, who brought me a huge smiley face flower balloon. Not only did it bring a smile to my face to see and visit with them, but the balloon brought smiles to the faces of the people I met in the hallways and lobby as I made my way out to the car to go home. The balloon continues to make me smile as I look at it clipped to an arrangement in our living room. It was a very thoughtful gesture. Thank you, Mary and Jane!

I am down to seven treatments left, and with the help of my new medication for nerve damage, I have regained some of the feeling in my lips, fingers, and toes. Hopefully, with continued use of the medication, I will regain the feeling in the rest of my lips and tongue. Muscle, bone, and joint aches continue to be part of my life, all side effects of the third chemo drug. It feels like a bad case of the flu each day, and I take medication to try to help me cope with those symptoms as well. Positive thoughts, positive results, right?

Against all odds, I have also lost four pounds in the past two weeks. And no, I have not been dieting. I have just been trying to eat sensibly and not to worry too much about the impending weight gain I have been predicted to see. I just want to beat the breast cancer and then worry about getting rid of the extra weight once I am healthy. Talk about patience being a virtue, especially when clothing choices are limited and shoes don't fit on your feet due to swelling. Hopefully, this too shall pass!

My mom's left eye continues to improve, but she is slated for monthly eye injections to help improve her vision and to keep the eye stable from wet macular degeneration.

So when I get up each morning and I am still thinking rationally for the most part and can get dressed and drive to work, I am satisfied and feel blessed that I have remained as stable as I have through this ordeal. I once again say "Thank you" to the countless people who have supported me through cards, messages, phone calls, visits, remembrances, prayers, and thinking of me. In other words, they just plainly walk by my side. The journey continues better than I had anticipated. I know I have God and all of you to thank for that being the case. You have been incredible. Love you!

Tuesday, September 6, 2011, 7:51 p.m., CDT

Down to Six

I finished my tenth chemo session just before noon today, so I am down to six treatments left. Slowly but surely, I have been working my way through each week, hoping and praying that I will be able to continue to work full time and stay in a positive environment. There is no doubt that time goes by much more quickly when you are productive and focusing on the future rather than dwelling on the present.

I did visit personally with Dr. Panwalkar this morning about how best to manage my ongoing pain, quite literally throughout my whole body, a normal side effect of this third chemo, and, more specifically, lower back pain causing some leg spasms. I also have ongoing nerve damage. Some has gotten better with medication; other areas are just starting to show up. Dr. Panwalkar has suggested, as I get closer to finishing my chemo, I may have to work more hours from home so I can rest in between the work time I am putting in. My mind is functioning well, but my body is having other ideas.

Thankfully, my boss and I were aware that I would need to rest more coming into the end of my chemo treatments. It is just hard for me to give up ground of going to the office each day outside of Tuesday, my chemo day. So Dr. Panwalkar has suggested that I work at the office while I am able physically and then potentially transition to every other day as I need to rest more. It wasn't what I wanted to hear today, but I understand I need to do what is in my best interest as a cancer patient.

Several people took the time to send me some encouraging gifts over the past few days, not to mention cards and e-mails. Thank you for continuing to walk with me on my journey. If it seems long to you, you can't imagine how it feels to me. Just know that I make it a point as I encounter others who have recently been diagnosed with cancer to tell them to have patience and perseverance and, most especially, to think positively. That mental prescription has worked well for me so far.

My family continues to be a special source of strength, getting me to appointments, calling or personally visiting to make certain I am doing well, encouraging me when I am not positive, and inviting me out for an occasional dinner when I feel up to it. I know I don't say it often enough, but thank you so much for all you have done. I love you!

Finally, I count on all of your continuing prayers as I get through each week. To everyone who has been with me on this journey, thank you. I appreciate you and feel most fortunate to have you all in my life. Love you!

Wednesday, September 14, 2011, 6:15 a.m., CDT

And Then There Were Five

That is right. I am down to five chemo sessions left after yesterday. I had a great visit with Dr. Panwalkar prior to my chemo session. He answered some questions about when my port could be removed after the sessions were completed. The answer? As soon as I wanted. That was like music to my ears because I have not been able to sleep lying on my right side, my favorite position before the port was implanted. Another thing to look forward to in a few weeks!

Yesterday, Dr. Panwalkar brought forward the possibility of participating in another clinical trial, which involves a drug that has been shown to prevent the reoccurrence of breast cancer. I would take the medication twice a day for a five-year period. We will discuss the pros and cons of my participation as I get closer to finishing my chemo treatments. Just know that, if there is a chance that I could participate in something that not only helps me but could help others down the line, then I will give it serious consideration.

We also talked about what I should anticipate going into the daily radiation treatments, which will most likely start mid-November and last six weeks rather than the five I was hoping for. Oh, well. I will just have to be brave and endure those treatments with the same positive, forward-looking attitude that has been my saving grace through chemo sessions so far. Hopefully by the end of the year, I will have made it through all of the medical procedures prescribed to battle my breast cancer and I can start the New Year with a new lease on life.

I continue to work full time. I know some people are thinking, "Is she out of her mind?" The answer is no. By working, I am the beneficiary of a positive, giveback environment, wherein I interact with caring, compassionate people, both at the office and those I meet as volunteers, business partners, and people we are serving. It amazes me each day that, when I wake and get ready for work, I feel fatigued and achy, but by the time I get to the office or, in some instances, do work from home, just doing positive, productive work makes me feel so much better. I then know I can survive this ordeal. If that is called living for work, then I guess that is true, especially now.

I want to share that, over the past week, I have met with a number of people who have told me that they continue to pray for me. Just hearing those words and knowing in my heart that they are true means the world to me. It has been a long journey over the past few months. At times, inside I wondered if I were going to make it to the end, but knowing so many people were pulling and praying for me gave me the strength to continue on.

I also realize that, when you hear from someone who is going through this type of a challenge, it is more comforting when he or she talks in positive terms and with a sense of humor. So I have embraced that philosophy and tried to live my life in that manner through my cancer fight. Thank you for being so strong and encouraging through these many months. I know I still have a ways to go, but I look forward to the next few months, knowing that God is with me and you too are all walking with me. That gives me the courage to battle on until I complete my journey.

To those people who have been recently diagnosed with cancer or have just undergone surgery and are looking at starting chemo or radiation, remember to stay strong and positive and focus on looking to the future. So many people are praying for you. Along with God's loving embrace, they will help carry you through what lies ahead.

Finally, a friend sent a wonderful e-mail yesterday, which included the following line: "Life is important like people we know who are special, and so we keep them close ... Live today because tomorrow is not promised." The e-mail also talked about how important it is to say "I love you" while you have the chance. So to my family, friends, and all who have been by my side, just know how much I love you and thank you for being with me through my life and, most especially, this cancer battle. I will never forget your compassion, prayers, and love.

Wednesday, September 21, 2011, 6:46 a.m., CDT

Digging down Deep

Jill came into the kitchen yesterday morning and said to me, "After this morning, you will be down to four chemo sessions left." And I looked at her and said, "And the end can't come soon enough." My patience, willpower, resolve, bravery, courage, and positive thinking have been tested through this journey. I came home from chemo yesterday feeling pretty good, made it through the evening doing okay, and then had a rough night last night. No matter which way I tried to sleep, I felt heaviness in my chest that just would not go away. But somehow, I persisted, prayed, and slept a few hours.

When I swung my legs over the side of the bed this morning and sat up, I thought, "Do I have enough energy to get up and go to work?" I checked my pulse, and it was strong. I stretched and did not feel a great deal of pain, just the normal overall achiness that accompanies treatments with this type of chemo drug. I took some great big, deep breaths. Slowly, I stood up and started to feel a little better. All the time, I was talking to myself, saying, "You can do it. Just take small steps."

I made my way to the kitchen to peel an orange, something I have done nearly every day since I was diagnosed. And on the days I didn't eat an orange, I drank some orange juice. For anyone going through this type of battle, you do not want to come down with a cold, any other type of flu symptoms, or respiratory illness, so persist in eating an orange each morning to get yourself off to a good start. So many "bugs" are out in the world that develop in the fall and winter. I always pray that people keep that in mind for the folks with depressed immune systems who cannot afford to catch an illness. I plan to drive to work this morning. It will keep me positive and focused on the future.

As I rested yesterday, with our family friend, Pat, who lived in Cando for many years and recently moved to the Fargo area, faithfully watching over me, I smiled, feeling blessed and grateful when I thought about a few of the ways people reached out to me recently.

Pat was by my side to make certain no health issues cropped up following my chemo treatment. She and Mom have been in contact because, if Mom could not be here, she was determined that someone she knew well would be by my side following treatments so Jill could go back to work. Moms have a way of taking care of things, even if they are a distance away. I love you, Mom!

My cousin's wife is eating different forms of chocolate on my behalf (or so she says), and being a cancer survivor herself, she has consistently sent encouraging e-mails. A friend called to say when he was walking his dog the other day that he heard geese flying overhead and thought of me and the Cando area with hunting season starting, and throughout our conversation, he told me how strong I had been through my battle so far and how proud he was of me.

During several meetings at the office, I have received hugs, encouraging words, a kiss on the cheek, a touch on the arm, or thoughtful notes on my desk. A chocolate bar was dropped off at the office, fruit slices were delivered in person, flowers were brought over with a catering order, eating establishment coupons appeared on my desk, and several people shared garden produce recently.

My coworkers ask if they can do something to help me with my work, or they quite simply just do a task that would take me twice as long as normal to do now. And the many people who e-mail and I talk to continue to offer encouragement and prayers and ask how they can help make my journey easier. The generosity of spirit and compassion demonstrated at this point in my battle takes my breath away. It confirms to me the very best in the people who surround me as

I walk this path. How do I even begin to say "Thank you" to everyone? Just know I am holding you all close to my heart.

A few journal entries and e-mails ago, I spoke about the big smiley face with bright pink petals flower balloon that several friends brought to me during a chemo session. The balloon has been quite the character. As it has aged gracefully, we have video of it trying to watch TV while a breeze blows it about. We have watched it slowly dropping closer to the floor as the helium depletes, and yesterday, it seemed to reach out to me as I waited patiently for Jill to get home from work. It was as if it were saying, "You are not alone." No, I promise I am not imagining things. It just confirms what comfort a smiley face can bring to you through a grin on the face of a loved one, nurse, friend, or total stranger. A smile is a powerful thing!

So, four more chemo sessions to go. I pray that God continues to bless me with stamina, courage, a continued sense of humor, and health, as good as it can be right now. I thank him for the many blessings he has already bestowed upon me, including your friendship and support. Thank you for your continued prayers. I love you all for being with me as I completed phase I and my surgery, approached the close of phase II and my chemo treatments, and prepare for phase III and my radiation treatments. Day by day, step by step, all in good time, we will get there together. Love you!

Tuesday, September 27, 2011, 12:40 p.m., CDT

Focused and Reaching for the End of Chemo

When you endure something like what I am going through, the smaller the number, which is now three chemo sessions, the more anxious you become. You long to be able to move the clock forward. You visualize the time when your life hopefully becomes more normal, like:

- Being able to take the extra nutritional supplements you have been longing for since April

- Being able to sleep on your right side at night

- Washing your hair and having to work with it so it looks just right

- Plucking your eyebrows because you now have them back

- Walking up and down stairs (or just plain walking for that matter) without the spasms and exhaustion that overcome you a few steps into the stroll

It amazes me what people take for granted every single day, and this includes me as well. Most of us wake up each morning being able to open our eyes, feeling our heart beating, stretching and knowing our brain and muscles are working, and knowing that our senses are fully functioning. Thousands in the world who surround us have their senses profoundly affected by a disease that they will battle for the rest of their lives. When I start feeling sorry for myself going through this cancer fight, I try to remember how very fortunate I am to still have complete use of all of my senses. Yes, some have been diminished during this ordeal, but I have been reassured that, because of my age and after chemo treatments, most should be restored. On the more challenging days, I try to remember the difficulties that other people are getting through, and my issues and how I address them seem much more doable. I try to remember that I "CAN-DO" it. (I really do love my hometown and the name that has given me strength through my journey.)

Once again this past week, I was reminded that countless people are praying for me during my battle, and I was humbled when my journal was used anonymously as a source of education and inspiration for the hundreds of people placed in a situation similar to mine. I know I have alluded to the fact that people are comforted when someone they are concerned about approaches an illness, such as mine, with dogged determination, a will to win the fight, staying positive and focused on the future. Perhaps that resonated with the folks who listened to my journal entries being read. To them, I was an anonymous woman diagnosed with breast cancer who was battling to regain her health back and, ultimately, her life. For me, granting access to my journal entries was a way to give back in gratitude to God and all of you for how well my cancer battle has unfolded. I also wanted to give hope to those fighting their own cancer battle and, hopefully, encourage those who will be diagnosed in the future with the knowledge that they too can walk this path and win.

Family becomes especially important at times like these, and mine has been by my side through this fight from day one. We have learned not to take life for granted. That most likely is because this is not the first time that cancer has made its presence known in our immediate family, and we know all too well what effect that type of fight has on a family. My oldest brother Fred lost his battle with brain cancer after a four-year fight back in the early seventies. And other battles have been waged on both sides of my family with various types of cancers. My diagnosis, however, was the first for breast cancer in my family. So, awareness and vigilance has been a new source of concern for my family members. Hopefully, we will not have another one of us fighting this battle in the future, but if so, we will have greater knowledge to win.

To those of you who shared your cancer battle stories with me recently, thank you. Know that your courage will inspire me and give me hope as I continue my journey in the months ahead. To those of you, who continue to remember me through your thoughtful gestures and prayers, please know how fortunate and blessed I feel to know you are by my side and in this battle with me. Rest assured that I will stay focused and reach for the end, all in the hopes of a positive outcome. There is no rest for the weary. It's simply victory ahead! Love you!

Tuesday, October 4, 2011, 2:15 p.m., CDT

Never a Dull Moment

As I was cruising through the week, or so I thought, following my last chemo session, I all of a sudden started feeling a little more lethargic and out of it on Wednesday evening. When I woke up on Thursday morning, my hands, feet, and ankles were, as I lovingly call it, "poufy." So I called Andrea. Laughter and then some tears filled our conversation. I told her how grateful I was for her being on the other end of the phone, not only now, but throughout my cancer battle. I said I felt something wasn't quite right with how I was feeling.

After some discussion, it was decided I should take some medication to try to pull off some of the fluid weight I was accumulating. So when I hung up the phone, I took the prescribed medication I had on hand, and within about a half hour, I started experiencing severe muscle spasms. So I took prescribed medication to relax my muscles. I drove to work, and by 1:00 p.m., I was not doing very well, so I drove back home and called Andrea to update her.

Meanwhile, our family friend, Pat, came to sit with me, at the request of my mom who has been back in Cando, two hundred miles away. Around 2:00 p.m., Dr. Panwalkar's office called, requesting I go to the walk-in clinic because of the concern about the fluid weight gain and my blood pressure. So Pat drove me to the walk-in clinic, where I wore a mask to protect against other illnesses, and I was seen fairly quickly. After confirming I had gained six pounds in less than two days and finishing some lab work and three chest X-rays, I was sent on my way, along with Jill, who came to sit with me, with four additional prescriptions/over-the-counter drugs to get me back on my feet. As you may have heard me say, "Never a dull moment!"

I made it through the week and weekend, a few pounds lighter from the fluid coming off me, and I've been trying to rest to regain strength and energy for this week and my chemo session this morning. I had a blood draw first thing Monday morning, and I saw Dr. Panwalkar this morning at 8:15 a.m., followed by my chemo session at 9:15 a.m. I am now down to two sessions left, and my patience will be tested as never before trying to get through these next two weeks.

As many of you know, it is Breast Cancer Awareness Month, and a flourish of pink is being seen everywhere—from players in the NFL wearing pink, to manufacturers offering a percentage back for various breast cancer programs and research, to a number of awareness walks being held. I can honestly say I have never been more in tune with their efforts than this year, being right in the middle of my battle. So if you have an opportunity to support any endeavor that will help someone you love perhaps in the future or, God forbid, yourself, please step up and do it. Thousands of women and men would sincerely appreciate your help. Hopefully, someday soon we will have a cure for cancer, in whatever form it appears.

A friend of mine forwarded an e-mail recently that focused on a penny. I know I may have mentioned to some of you somewhere along the way that my dad used to have me pick up the pennies we would find either cleaning motel rooms, walking across a parking lot, or on a sidewalk. He always told me I might need the penny someday.

I have found quite a few pennies over the course of my lifetime since my dad passed away and a number fairly recently since my diagnosis and treatment. I hold close to my heart the knowledge my dad, one of my angels, is in this fight with me, along with my brother, grandparents, aunts, uncles, cousins, and dear friends who have departed this world before me. I also know that God and all of you are walking with me, too. The peace and calm that brings to my life is beyond measure, as is the gratitude I feel knowing you are all part of my life. Thank you for your vigilance, commitment, love, and prayers for me during this long ordeal.

So it is two more chemo treatments to go in phase II and then on to phase III in mid-November. Slow and steady will win this race, and I am pacing myself to cross the finish line in victory. Love you!

Tuesday, October 11, 2011, 1:45 p.m., CDT

Erring on the Side of Caution

During last week's appointment with Dr. Panwalkar, he discovered a sore spot/lump on the outside of my right breast. You may recall that my left breast had two tumors and a lymph node under my left arm was diagnosed with breast cancer in April. Dr. Panwalkar, Jill, and I discussed how important it was to monitor the area, and if it continued to be an issue, we would potentially schedule an ultrasound to make certain we erred on the side of caution and that there was no additional breast cancer that we needed to address.

We also discussed that I would have my port removed early morning on October 25. I would see Dr. Panwalkar following the removal, and then I would have my initial visit with Dr. Ethan Foster, my radiation oncologist later that day. The appointment with Dr. Foster is to start planning for all the facets included in my six weeks of radiation treatments, tentatively scheduled to begin November 14.

As I progressed through the week and weekend, I just kept praying and asking God to spare me from further breast cancer. When I continued to feel the soreness and lump Monday morning, I reached out to Andrea and asked her to speak with Dr. Panwalkar for his advice. By 4:00 p.m. on Monday, Andrea had called back to schedule an ultrasound of the affected area to make certain we knew if anything needed additional treatment. I hope it is just another sore spot due to the chemo treatments, similar to what I experienced in the right breast several weeks ago, just in a different spot.

I completed my fifteenth chemo session late this morning, and I will have an ultrasound on the right breast at 2:15 p.m. today to see if we need to address anything further before my port is removed on October 25th. I do not want to have the port removed and then find out I am dealing with additional breast cancer on the right side, which would probably necessitate reinsertion of the port.

As I have mentioned previously, we are erring on the side of caution, which will give me and many other people praying for me better peace of mind. So if you have extra prayers to offer up on my behalf, I would sincerely appreciate them. I know God will not give me any more than I can handle, and I know he and all of you have been by my side so far and I will make it through it, no matter what lies ahead.

I know many women (and men) who have shared their stories about a second breast cancer diagnosis that continue to do well. I will pray that I am nearing the end of my chemo sessions with no further worries and I will move forward into my radiation treatments as scheduled. I will also remember the stories of success following a second diagnosis as I wait for my test results.

Until then, I will count on your continued thoughts and prayers as I look at completing my chemo treatments next Tuesday, October 18. Thanks for being by my side during this worrisome time. Love you.

Tuesday, October 11, 2011, 4:28 p.m., CDT

Needle Biopsy Tomorrow ... Keep Those Prayers Coming!

First, thank you, Jill, for getting me through my chemo session this morning, and Pat, our dear friend from Cando, now a West Fargo resident, for getting me to my appointment this afternoon. An ultrasound scan was performed on a sore spot and lump located on the outside portion of my right breast today at 2:15 p.m.

When the technician completed the scan, she asked the radiologist to join us in the procedure room to review the results. Once again, she indicated that, because of my heavy, dense breast tissue, it was difficult getting a clear scan of the area of concern. So she asked that a needle biopsy of the area be performed tomorrow morning at 11:15 a.m., in the hopes that I would have a definitive answer regarding the tissue sample by Friday of this week.

I want you all to know that the radiologist seemed much more upbeat today, compared to her demeanor when she consulted on the ultrasound scans and performed the needle biopsies back in April. She and Dr. Panwalkar are erring on the side of caution, and for that, I am grateful. Hopefully by Friday, we will all breathe a sigh of relief, but if not, I have no doubt in my mind that I will make it through whatever lies ahead.

Thank you for continuing to keep me in your prayers, especially for good results on this new area of concern. I love you so much for hanging in there with me during the last few months. I am so very grateful for the ongoing support, well-wishes, remembrances, and prayers. As soon as I hear something on Friday, I will send an update. Love you.

Thursday, October 13, 2011, 4:45 p.m., CDT

The Phone Call Just Came In

And the biopsy taken of tissue in the right breast has come back as normal. That is, there is no further breast cancer in the area of concern. When the nurse said she was calling from Dr. Panwalkar's office, I held my breath and just listened. And then the tears started to well in my eyes from the relief and joy in knowing God had granted our prayers. I could not help knowing that countless prayers were being offered up on my behalf. I had such a sense of peace and calm on the inside. However, after having received the news I did in April and going through what I have so far, I have learned never to take anything for granted until I have a definitive answer, and this time around, it was great news.

My family was so relieved for me when I called them to share the good news this time, as were my boss and coworkers. Being euphoric at a time when I have been through fifteen chemo treatments with one left to go and then six weeks of radiation still in my future seems a bit strange. But if you talk with anyone who has walked this path, just having an answer that is more definitive and also positive in a good way takes on way more significance than you can put into words. It is called peace of mind.

One of my family members said, "Yay for our team!" and I could not agree more. I have been so very fortunate and blessed to have you all with me on my journey and all on my team. Thank you for praying for me over the last six-plus months and offering up the extra prayers for a good test result. I know that, when I say my prayers tonight, I will thank God for my good news. I will pray for those who did not get good news today in their cancer battle and ask that he walk by their side as they battle their way back to better health. Thanks for joining me in offering a similar prayer.

So I will prepare for my final chemo session next Tuesday, October 18, and I will rejoice in knowing I will move on to phase III of my journey. Thank you, God! Love you.

Tuesday, October 18, 2011, 12:45 p.m., CDT

Phase II Completed!

Chemo session sixteen has been successfully finished. Phase II is complete. Am I rejoicing? You bet I am. I am rejoicing in:

- My recent good news on the second breast cancer biopsy

- Knowing I hopefully will not lose any more feeling in my toes, feet, fingers, hands, lips, and tongue due to nerve damage

- The fact I will soon be able to taste food that is not just cold or hot but actually has flavor

- Already having the hair on my head growing back, albeit almost all snow-white (I actually had my hair trimmed this past Saturday. Thank you, Lacey.)

- Regaining my stamina and strength for the time being because the chemo drugs are not killing off good cells along with the bad ones

- Working in the office on Tuesdays because I haven't had to endure a chemo session on that day

- Refraining from saying to Jill that I can't wait for the chemo to be done so I don't ache all over

- Being able to sleep on my right side once my port is removed

- And other things much too long to list here

Have these experiences blessed me so far? There is no doubt. Jill might not feel the same way after I had a complete meltdown Sunday morning. I nearly fell backward down a flight of stairs at our condo after stubbornly trying to carry up a load of laundry from our basement laundry room. I was scared, frustrated, and, quite honestly, at the end of my rope with this whole ordeal. I have tried to live my life as positively and normally as possible, enduring through all of the procedures, surgeries, chemo treatments, appointments, my job, and chores at home.

Jill took the brunt of my tirade Sunday morning with hurt tears in her eyes. She picked up the pieces of my broken spirit and reminded me that she told me up front she might not be my best caregiver. But nothing could be farther from the truth. She has been with me for fifteen of the sixteen chemo sessions, my surgery, and every day of my journey. How do you say thank you to someone that devoted who has made me laugh about the most challenging things, who has come into my room each morning to check to see how I am doing, and who has reminded me that things could be worse? Obviously yelling would not be the right way, but hopefully she knows I will be by her side should she have challenges ahead. I love you, Jill. You have been awesome!

I will have little time to celebrate the end of chemo treatments because next Tuesday, October 25, I have:

- Removal of my port

- A follow-up appointment with Dr. Panwalkar, including a flu shot

- An afternoon appointment with Dr. Foster to gear up for my six weeks of daily radiation treatments, tentatively scheduled to begin on November 14

Phase III, here I come!

As a breast cancer survivor, the flourish of pink so visible during this Breast Cancer Awareness Month is gratifying. I am so very proud of all of the efforts focused on education, research, encouragement, celebrating victories, and remembering those who fought the good fight but lost their battle. The stories of people who walked this path before me resonate deep within me and, I am certain, touch hundreds of others currently fighting the battle. To those participating, thank you! I hope that those diagnosed in the future know a large army of survivors is available to reach out to for advice, encouragement, compassion, and love. Remember, you will not be alone. I know that first-hand.

So to all of you patiently waiting and praying for the successful completion of my chemo treatments, we made it. I am elated, and I will thank God for his blessings poured down upon me and for you all being part of my life. I would appreciate your continued prayers as I undergo the port removal procedure next week and then head into phase III of my journey. Thank you so much. Love you!

RADIATION

Wednesday, October 26, 2011, 8:29 a.m., CDT

Port Is Out ... Phase III Started

Monday was a tough day emotionally for me. I was very apprehensive about how my port was going to be removed. I have been through numerous surgeries, procedures, biopsies, and scans, over the past few years without being under (so to speak), including three nose surgeries to rebuild the left side of my nose following a Mohs procedure to remove basal cell carcinoma (skin cancer). So the thought of one more procedure, like having my port removed, without anesthesia, was about more than I could take, especially now.

In good news, I had a wonderful doctor who talked to me with compassion and understanding regarding my fears before, during, and after the port removal procedure yesterday morning. I was so grateful that he took time to recognize me as a person rather than just another patient in for another procedure. Even though I am quite sore today, I am happy the port is out and I don't have to deal with the ongoing neck spasms.

My appointment with Dr. Panwalkar went very well yesterday. He has allowed me to go back on my green tea. Yay! Hopefully that will help me get rid of some of the fluid I have been retaining. I can only hope. He answered multiple questions I had following my care after chemo. He was patient and thoughtful and maintained his sense of humor through all the questions, for which I was grateful. I did find out that it will take up to six months to regain most of my taste bud function and, hopefully, salvage feeling in my toes, feet, hands, fingers, lips, and tongue from nerve damage. It is a slow process, but he felt, because of my age, there was a good chance I would recover feeling in most, if not all, of the affected areas. I am grateful and will try to stay patient.

Dr. Panwalkar asked why I wasn't wearing my wig. I told him, because my hair was growing so well, I thought I did not need a wig anymore. I did place a photo of my Uncle Rich and me out in the photos section of my webpage so people can see that it is coming back. Progress in the right direction!

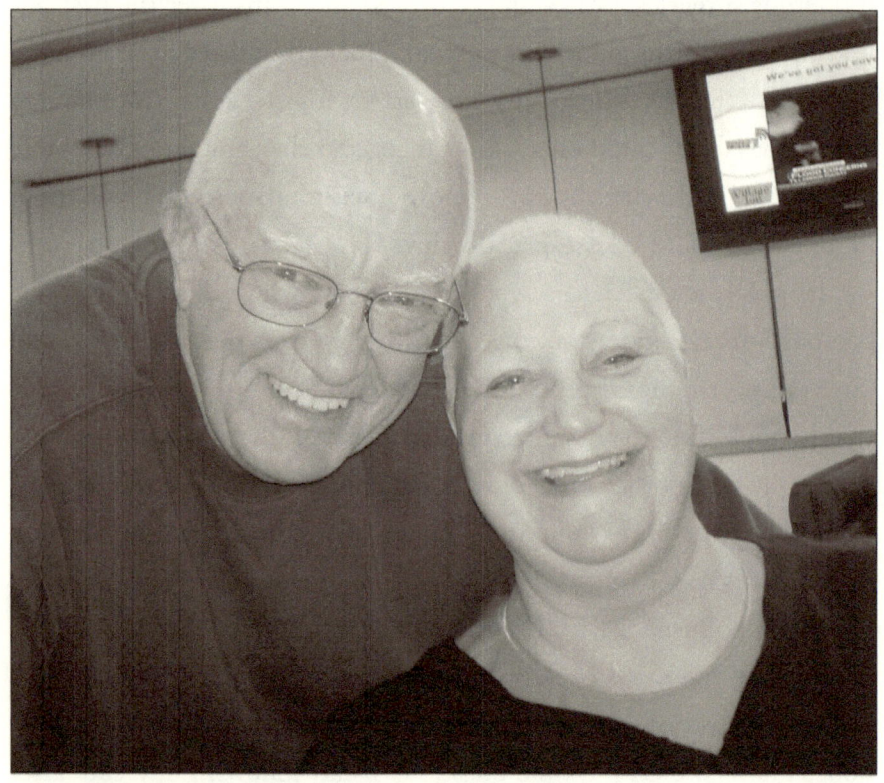

Birds of a feather flock together! That is the saying that came to mind when I saw the photo taken of my Uncle Richard and me as my hair started to grow back. He consoled me by saying at least mine was going to grow back!

I also had a chance to meet Dr. Foster and his nurse, Heather, yesterday afternoon, just two of a large contingent of providers for phase III. That appointment lasted about one and a half hours because we had so much to discuss regarding the six-plus weeks of daily radiation treatments. I will undergo a total of thirty-three treatments during this phase. With the hope of beginning on November 14, the initial scan and tattoo procedure has been scheduled for 9:30 a.m. this morning because a portion of the test and planning takes between seven to ten days to be returned prior to me starting radiation.

I am happy to report that I drove myself to my appointment this morning. It was a little challenging making some turns with my chest being sore, but I managed. I met with another nurse this morning, then went through the scan and tattooing procedure, and finished with a flu shot, which Dr. Panwalkar ordered, before heading out the door and driving home.

I have been told the most challenging health issues with radiation are fatigue and potential skin challenges. These treatments, like chemo, also have a cumulative effect, so the more treatments I endure, the more challenging the issues. There are also other potential side effects, although very minimal chances of damage/scarring of breast, lung, and heart tissue and secondary cancers due to the radiation treatments.

You listen, think through what it is that your medical team and you are trying to accomplish with the treatments, and then forge bravely ahead with the process. Persistence, patience, trust, and a positive attitude will again come into play. I pray that God will grant me all of those things, plus peace and calm for the next two-plus months. So I will drive to the cancer center Monday through Friday, with the exception of holidays, for six weeks and then hopefully to work following each treatment.

Donna, our next-door neighbor, thoughtfully put up a display last week celebrating the end of my chemo treatments, which greeted Jill and me when we opened our door to head out for work. What a thoughtful surprise from a dear friend. Thank you!

A box with some celebratory remembrances also arrived from my brother and sister-in-law and their family in South Carolina. It is always so challenging when you live a distance away and a family member is undergoing this type of a journey. It reminds you never to take anything for granted and to be grateful for the thoughtfulness of the people who are in your life and walking by your side. Thank you!

Be it a card, guestbook entry, remembrance, e-mail, positive comment, helpful deed, phone call, prayer chain, rosary, individual prayer, and asking that a mass be read on my behalf, among other things, it is such a comfort knowing I am not alone in this fight. Thank you all for everything you have done to make this journey easier. I am grateful.

So, God willing, I will continue to prepare for the next phase of my journey and the start of radiation. I would sincerely appreciate your continued thoughts and prayers. Love you!

Friday, November 4, 2011, 8:02 a.m., CDT

Building Resolve and Courage

Since Wednesday of last week, I have been rejoicing in the fact that I do not have to endure further chemo treatments and I just get to rest (so to speak) in between what I have just been through and what lies ahead. I have made it a point to continue to work full time at my job, and I have tried to work in a few other things around the condo I have put on hold since I started this battle. If you would talk with my mom, Jill, or any of my coworkers about how I have been doing, they would most likely tell you I have talked a lot about my "poufy" feet and toes, "cankles," legs, and hands and how achy I continue to be and the extreme fatigue I have been feeling.

Even though I have worked to remove as much salt from my diet as possible and have been taking medication to reduce the fluid I am retaining, Dr. Panwalkar has told me that the fluid retention is a side effect of the chemo treatments I have been through and partially due to the flu shot I had last Wednesday. Evidently I will continue to feel this way for several more days before I turn the corner and head in a better direction. Are we there yet?

I have to smile and laugh on the inside when people finally get a chance to see me in person. Their first reaction is to comment on how well my hair is growing back, albeit mostly snow-white, but growing fairly fast. Then they want to touch it to see what it feels like, and some actually rub my head. Because I am so grateful my hair is returning, their actions and joy make me happy. Every small step, every expression of support is a blessing.

The area where my port was removed is healing nicely, and I am thrilled to report that I have been sleeping a portion of the night on my right side. It is comforting and a step back toward normalcy for me. Yippee!

The generosity of compassionate hearts continues to lift me up along my journey. A box of everything pink, with breast cancer awareness being the main theme, arrived from our business supply vendor. A mass was offered up in my name, chocolate treats to keep me going were shared with me, a cheerful, singing phone call was received, and a call to ask if Jill and I wanted to go for dinner was appreciated. My cousin changed his travel path on the way to an appointment when he saw me in my vehicle with pink ribbons flying from the rearview mirrors and soft, pink hat on my head just to see how I was doing. And I continued to receive messages of encouragement delivered in person, through a friend, or by e-mail or card. Each action reaches deep within me to lift me up and keep me going.

I share this information in my updates because so many have asked what they can do in this type of a situation. They have asked how they can help their loved one or friend. All the many gestures over the past six-plus months are, quite simply, priceless because they have come from people who want nothing more than to have me win this fight and to be healthy and whole again. Rest assured I am fighting with all I am to make that happen.

So I am building my resolve and courage to tackle radiation during this lull in my treatment plan. I stay snuggled under the covers each morning just a little while longer, asking God to give me the inner peace and strength to endure what lies ahead and thanking him for how well things have gone so far and the countless people cheering and praying me through to the finish line. Thanks for being by my side with your continued support and prayers. You and your actions have been blessings in my life. Love you.

Wednesday, November 9, 2011, 7:49 a.m., CST

Waiting for the Call

I know for a fact that I don't have enough patience. I know that, as a middle-aged woman, I am supposed to have lots of it by now. But I still feel like a kid on the inside, and waiting to hear from Dr. Foster's office with a confirmation start date and time has me feeling helpless and anxious.

I admit it. I am a control freak. If I have a plan and can work toward delivering it successfully, I am happy to take the steps to finish the task. I also know I want my course of radiation treatments to be the most effective they can be, and I realize many other patients are either getting started, in the middle of, or finishing their radiation treatments as well. Patience, Cindy. Patience!

Keep in mind that my goal, mentally and physically, is focused on completing my radiation treatments by December 31. I have counted out the thirty-three days it will take me to complete my treatments on the calendar, using Monday through Friday as potential days of treatment. I have accounted for one day for the Thanksgiving holiday, one for the Christmas holiday, and no weekend dates. If I do not start on November 14, I will not complete my treatments by the end of this calendar year. Will that be the end of the world? No. But I set a goal in my mind, and I hope to fulfill it.

Why would anyone long to start a treatment plan like this any sooner than possible? I will admit that I feel like a prisoner most days, counting the days until I am free of medical tests, procedures, and treatments, that is, when I can call my life my own once again. I have written about how I long for normalcy in my life, how I can't wait to be able to just do my job without working around my medical appointments. You can bet I will never take being healthy for granted again. Nor will I ever forget the people who so consistently and graciously lift me up when I feel overwhelmed. That applies to my home and work life.

I am an independent woman. I try to tackle things and be responsible for my work and self on my own. So over the past seven months, the hardest thing I have had to do is rely on other people to help me. Being capable and independent is who I am and who I will always be. However, God has made me a more humble person through my journey. I have had to reach out and request assistance. I may grit my teeth and not be happy about it, but I have done what I needed to do. For those of you who have helped me understand that it is okay to ask for assistance and who have assisted me or tried, thank you.

I am still focusing on the positive, which includes completing a wonderful follow-up appointment with Dr. Bouton yesterday. We had a great give-and-take conversation. My surgical site looks good, and he has assured me that, with patience, I will hopefully recover most of the feeling under my left arm and breast. I will go back to see him in April 2012, following my next mammogram. He is reassuring and a genuinely nice person. His presence in my life has blessed me.

So I am waiting for the call, and I ask you continue your prayers for my patience and a successful completion of my journey over the next two months. Thank you.

Persistent? Check. Positive? Check. Patient? Working on it! Love you? No doubt about it!

Friday, November 11, 2011, 12:00 p.m., CST

Date and Time for Phase III Start Confirmed

I will start my radiation treatments on Monday evening, November 14, at 5:50 p.m. Even though I had been hoping to take the minutes at our quarterly board meeting on Monday evening at 6:15 p.m. and to say "Thank you" to our board members for their tremendous support through my breast cancer journey so far, I will be doing what I need to do to get started on my radiation treatments and have this battle behind me, God willing, by the end of the year.

Initially when I spoke with the radiation scheduling department at around 6:00 p.m. last evening, they had me starting radiation on Tuesday, November 15, at 8:30 p.m., which would have had me carrying my thirty-third and final radiation treatment into next year. That was disappointing in a number of ways, but primarily from a mental standpoint. I desperately wanted to start the New Year with a renewed sense of health and well-being. I am most grateful that the person I was speaking with regarding my start date understood how important completing my radiation treatments by the end of the year was to me. She listened to me, told me she wanted to check a few things, and said she would call back. My spirits soared when she called back to tell me I would be starting on Monday rather than Tuesday so I could finish by the end of the year.

I am committed to getting through this fight in the best possible shape—mentally, spiritually, and physically—as I possibly can. Without the incredible support and prayers of an army of compassionate people and God's blessing, I would not be where I am today. I plan to tick off each radiation treatment one by one until I reach December 30 and complete this phase of my journey. Thanks for being by my side as we press through to the end and your love and prayers. Love you.

Thursday, November 17, 2011, 5:50 a.m., CST

Three Down … Thirty to Go

As I prepared the boardroom for our quarterly board meeting on Monday afternoon, I kept watching the clock. I knew I needed to pick my mom up at our condo before heading for my first radiation treatment, which was scheduled for 5:50 p.m. She wanted to go with me for my first treatment, not only for moral support, but also to have a chance to meet Dr. Foster. As the time grew closer to leaving the office, my stomach was in knots. I was moving into the third phase of my journey, and I prayed that all would go well.

We arrived at the cancer center shortly after 5:30 p.m. I dropped Mom off at the door, parked my vehicle, and walked to the front entrance. The building is in the midst of a large renovation project, so the front entrance has quite literally been moving over the course of several days. Mom had already struck up a conversation with Rose, the greeter in the evenings to let patients into the building, which otherwise would be closed. I also greeted Rose, who directed us down the hallway to the radiation department.

Four other patients, all with a family member accompanying them, were waiting for radiation treatment. All were different ages with a common theme, getting through treatment. It was comforting to see that they were smiling when they came out a door after finishing. Because of a widespread power outage in the Fargo-Moorhead area on Monday, the department had been delayed in moving patients through, so we patiently waited our turn until our names were called.

I introduced myself to Bonnie at the front desk. Bonnie and Jennifer are the first people you speak with when calling the radiation department, and both are obviously well suited for their jobs. Care and compassion are what you hear, and both demonstrate this. When thirty-three radiation treatments face you, you are grateful to observe those characteristics.

When my name was called around 7:00 p.m., I was asked to change clothes and to wait in an area that was quite literally a construction zone. What is heartening to see is that, no matter what the conditions of the building might be, the people tasked with completing your treatments are all continuing to do their jobs with a smile on their face.

One of the technicians came out to get me, and I walked down a long corridor to the radiation room. Two technicians worked to align me on the long, metal table. They worked with Dr. Foster to check alignments and came back in to reposition me again, and the process continued until the two red crosshairs were aligned exactly on my tattoos. At a point, I just closed my eyes and prayed for strength and the treatment to be over. After thirty-five minutes of lying as still as possible, with my left arm above my head and my right arm tucked under my body, I was done. I didn't have any discomfort from the radiation treatment itself during the session.

I hopped off the table, proceeded back to the dressing room, and got dressed. And when I entered the waiting room, I celebrated with Mom that I only had thirty-two treatments left. Dr. Foster's nurse weighed me. I had lost nine pounds from the previous time I had been weighed, and we proceeded to a brief office visit with Dr. Foster. I will see him every Monday so he can monitor how my body and, more specifically, the area being radiated are reacting.

We talked about how important the application of topical aloe vera gel three times per day to the area being treated would be for me. If the skin and tissue started to break down toward the end of the treatments, he would suggest other prescribed lotions I could use. He also indicated the chest wall just below my left breast and the folds under the breast and arm would most likely be the most affected areas from radiation. I will be vigilant to make certain I care for the area so I hopefully don't have any complications.

Mom and I were home by 8:30 p.m. Monday evening. The treatment times for the rest of the week are Tuesday at 8:20 p.m., Wednesday at 7:30 p.m., Thursday morning at 7:40 a.m., and Friday evening at 6:50 p.m. It's quite literally all over the clock, but whatever the times, I will be there to forge ahead.

On Tuesday evening, I met two other breast cancer patients. Both had endured chemo, which sounded very challenging compared to what I had been through. One had been hospitalized for six days following her first chemo, had lost her fingernails and toenails, and could only complete five out of six treatments because of severe nerve damage. The other had her challenges as well. I cried following treatment that night, out of complete gratefulness that God and all of you offering up prayers had helped carry me through my sixteen treatments with minimal side effects. A sense of guilt almost comes into play because I was so fortunate. Just know I recognize and appreciate that fact.

I will receive my radiation times for the following week on Friday, so my schedule will need to remain flexible to make certain I continue the process and work to complete my treatments by the end of the year. Thank you for your continued support and prayers, which will hopefully sustain me through this phase. Love you.

Tuesday, November 22, 2011, 12:18 p.m., CST

Giving Thanks

Thanksgiving, a time for giving thanks. And this year, more than any in the past, I have much for which to be thankful. My checkup appointments, reports, and procedures, all continue to go well. I am down to twenty-six radiation treatments, and they are going as anticipated. When I stepped on the scale last night for my weekly weigh-in, I was down another six pounds, a total of fifteen pounds over the past two weeks. Yes, they did ask if I were dieting, and no, I am not.

Dr. Panwalkar made me promise I would not diet until I had made it through my entire treatment schedule. I think the weight loss is due to a combination of things:

- Eating smarter and smaller portions

- Expending more energy in between chemo and radiation treatments while I had the stamina to move more

- Continuing my diuretic prescription

- Moving beyond the steroids that were part of my chemo treatments

Regardless of why, I know I feel better carrying less weight, and I will just be grateful for now.

Also at Dr. Panwalkar's request, I saw a physical therapist this morning to cope with the ongoing fluid retention in my feet, toes, ankles, and lower legs. She instructed I wear compression stockings and tennis shoes for the time being, do some ankle flexing exercises every half hour while sitting, and elevate my feet once I get home from work and more on the weekends.

I woke up Monday morning with five canker sores in my mouth. Dr. Foster said they are most likely a side effect of a highly depressed immune system, not my radiation treatments. As suggested, I have purchased an over-the-counter application that is working well. My hair, eyebrows, and eyelashes all continue to grow back. Pretty cool, especially when I get told my hair is starting to curl in places because it is so long (kidding, of course), but I am happy nonetheless.

I have continued to be scheduled for my radiation treatments right before one of the women I wrote about last week. She is close to my age, and we have much in common with our breast cancer battles. When I left the treatment room last evening, she was sitting in a chair waiting her turn. She stood up and walked toward me holding a beautiful silver necklace that held the breast cancer ribbon and a separate pink stone. She was wearing the same necklace. She looked me in the eyes and thanked me for helping calm her fears, making her feel at ease prior to her first radiation treatment, and leading by example. I started to cry and gave her a big hug because she had helped me in the same way. Her gesture was breathtaking.

At times, I wonder if I am worthy and why my journey has been so smooth and, for the most part, with little pain. Many times, I have been a reluctant participant in my walk, knowing I have no choice if I intend to win but trying to smile and be positive so my words and actions encourage those I meet or correspond with. I want everyone to know that I am committed to do all I need to do to regain my health.

So at this time of year, Thanksgiving, I offer up my thanks and praise to God for all of his blessings and to each of you for everything you have done on my behalf, for me, or in my name to get me this far in my breast cancer battle. May God bless all of you with health and happiness at this time of thanksgiving. I would appreciate you keeping me in your prayers. Thank you! Love you.

Wednesday, November 30, 2011 5:33 a.m., CST

Eleven Down … Twenty-two to Go!

That is right. I am one-third the way through my radiation treatments. I believe the saying is, "Time flies when you are having fun," and in my case, daily rather than weekly treatments are flying by. The receptionists and technicians greet me every day with a smile, and the nurses and Dr. Foster monitor my progress on a weekly basis.

My Monday morning visit with Dr. Foster went well. He is pleased with how the area being radiated appears and asked me to determine when I would work in a nap each day because my stamina was going to continue to be tested, and he knew I would become more fatigued as the treatments progressed. Suffice it to say, I have formulated a game plan for the daily nap request. I think I need to be more grateful that someone is actually asking me to do that each day. I know what you are thinking, "Where can I get that prescription?"

I stayed the same weight from last week at my weekly weigh-in. Not bad considering I celebrated the Thanksgiving holiday with my sisters, Jill and Vicki, and Tom, my brother-in-law. We had a wonderful meal and followed that up with a several-hour session of whist. Tom and I held our own against my two sisters. We each won one game of two. I felt sorry for Tom who would look at me and no doubt wonder, "Does she even know what she is doing at this point in time?" I know I granded several times where I looked at him and he just smiled and thought, "Here we go again." We had fun, and I was grateful for our time spent together.

Several days of leisurely rest and three meals a day followed up the holiday. Why do I feel so guilty just resting? Perhaps it is because I am not checking off the numerous things on the Cindy Eggl to-do list?

Note to self: Try to get over the fact that you were raised with a work ethic of "work before play" and the notion that "work is play."

I have now been fitted with my new compression stockings, which I will wear for two to three months depending on if my feet and ankles behave. I never realized how important it was to correctly fit and pull on this layer of footwear, but I do now. I have to admit that my legs felt much better last evening, so I will try to be a good kid and do what the doctor and physical therapist have ordered.

One of my favorite sayings keeps coming to mind, "Persistence pays off." That is true when I:

- Wake up each morning

- Eat my breakfast

- Get dressed

- Walk out to my vehicle in the cold morning air

- Drive to the cancer center while praying the roads are not slippery

- Park my vehicle and walk into the cancer center

- Say hello to the greeter at the door and the receptionist in the radiation area

- Have a chair to wait for my turn

- Change my clothes when I am called for my treatment

- Walk the hallway to the radiation room

- Greet the technicians

- Complete the fifteen- to twenty-minute treatment

- Tell everyone to have a great day and say I appreciate their work

- Proceed back to the dressing room

- Apply the aloe gel (the first of three to four times per day) to the area radiated

- Get dressed to head back out in the cold

- Smile when departing the cancer center because I have completed one more treatment

- Walk to my vehicle in prayer

- Drive to work

- Tackle my day

And now, I will do this daily routine with a nap included and pulling on my compression hose to boot. Surreal at this late stage of my battle? Yes, it is. My focus continues to be December 30, my final day of radiation treatments and to get there in the best physical, mental, and spiritual shape I can while trying to lead as normal a life as I can right now.

The people I have met on my breast cancer journey have profoundly changed my perspective on life. They have been all different ages and come from many different circumstances. But the common thread we have all had is:

- The initial fear when hearing the word "cancer"

- Determining a treatment plan with a wonderful medical team, kindnesses shown, a fighting spirit, and determination

- Staying the course to health through surgery and all the treatments and prayers

When you don't know what to do for someone in a health crisis, especially a long, drawn-out journey, pray. The calm and peace that it provides for both you and the recipient is healing. I know many prayers have blessed me. Thank you. I will continue to count on them to get me to December 30th and into the New Year with renewed health. Love you.

Sunday, December 4, 2011, 6:53 a.m., CST

Maintaining Dignity

It dawned on me on Friday when I finished my radiation treatment and I was asked if I would like a massage that many things in my life, and in particular, my health have changed since I heard the words, "You have breast cancer" on April 12. I always hesitate before saying yes to a massage because I don't know if my muscles will feel better or worse following the session. Gratefully, I have usually felt better, so I took them up on the offer, and I was glad I did.

You should solely base your decisions during a cancer battle on you winning the battle. Speaking from experience, a whole other side of your thought process simply wants you to maintain your dignity throughout the ordeal. You see, at least for me, that is where I have suffered the most at times over the past nine months.

The checklist goes like this:

- **Modesty.** Forget that. It goes out the window immediately when you know you will have to fight with every ounce of your being for your life. The medical team and those caring for you have to see your progress.

- **Appearance.** Well, let me think. For me, that has meant wearing jogging suits and comfortable clothes, whatever has been easiest to get on and off because my stamina has been severely tested and fatigue has been an issue. I have suffered the loss of my hair, eyebrows, eyelashes, and potentially a fingernail here or there. I don't have to worry about breast reconstruction, but thousands have and will.

- **Weight gain and bodily functions.** I don't have enough space to write at length about the indignities of these two issues, but clothing and shoes that do not fit anymore, feeling bloated constantly, making decisions about whether to take a product that helps with diarrhea or constipation on a daily basis, much less the gas that accompanies all of the medications you take, have made my life pretty interesting. Another irritating side effect includes a dry mouth that makes my lips stick to my teeth when talking. I drink lots of water to help, not to mention use special mouthwash, toothpaste, and gel to help control the breakdown of tissue and other bad side effects.

- **Dry skin.** You finally give up trying to slather on lotions. You are so tired that you rejoice in just being able to get through a shower as often as possible.

- **Skin and tissue breakdown from radiation treatments.** Time will tell. No perfumed body wash, metals in lotions, deodorant, or shaving is allowed.

- **Compression socks and tennis shoes.** I wear these to battle fluid retention and regain the health of my feet, toes, and legs for two to three more months. I can do that. I will count my blessings because I know I have fared much better than thousands of others who have walked this path.

- **Independence.** Good luck with this one. You really don't want to give up an inch of your independence, but you are forced to because of procedures, surgery, treatments, medication, and simply not being strong enough to care for yourself. The physical challenges can be humbling, but so can giving up your independence because you have to rely on others.

- **Confidence.** This characteristic is eroded almost immediately. You feel like your body has turned on you and you can never trust it again. But you must believe that you can overcome the challenge. You offer up your life to God and ask that he sees fit to get you through the battle and back to a place of normalcy. And you pray that others will help guide you and understand when you are weak, confused, lonely, or depressed or have gone round the bend, need assistance, or simply need to talk to get things out in an effort to regain your confidence.

- **Sense of humor.** Keep this one close to your heart. You cry, you laugh, you cry, and you laugh. And the laughter lifts the burden long enough for you to breathe and tell yourself one more time, "I am going to make it!"

- **Patience.** If you don't have it, you better get it because you will need every ounce that you can muster to get through this long and grueling ordeal. And you had better pray that your family, friends, coworkers, and folks you meet on a daily basis have it as well.

- **Faith.** It's such a pretty and powerful word. Without it, this journey will seem like it is insurmountable. You have to have faith in your medical team, family, and friends. You have to have faith that God will provide and not put you through more than you can handle and, most importantly, faith in yourself that you will not give up and will fight with all you are to win.

At times, I just need to write the things that I have held inside and thought about for months because I want others to know and appreciate how fortunate they are to have their health, and I hope they will continue to show compassion for those going through medical issues.

I am down to nineteen radiation treatments to get through. One at a time, I am persevering through to the end. Thank you for thinking of me, encouraging me, and praying for me on this long journey. I will count on your continued support and prayers until we reach the end. Love you.

Tuesday, December 13, 2011, 6:15 a.m., CST

The Path Becomes More Challenging

I am now down to thirteen radiation treatments left. As predicted, the first three-plus weeks went relatively without incident—just the tediousness of managing the daily routine, driving to the cancer center, and getting through each radiation treatment. The area being radiated has become more challenging. Swollen? Yes. Angry red in color? Yes. Painful? Yes. Skin challenges? Not yet, but some areas are getting thin like tissue paper. Am I worried about the next few weeks? Most definitely.

Following my treatment yesterday morning, I met with Dr. Foster and his nurse. I have been switched from aloe gel to Aquaphor, a Vaseline-like jelly to help with the severely sunburned look of the skin and to help the skin from breaking down any sooner than possible. I also have an area on my upper left back that the radiation treatment affects. The angle of the treatment is causing a red area. Jill has been applying aloe gel to that area before I go to bed at night. Thanks for the continuing care, Jill! In addition to the new jelly, it was also suggested that I purchase some men's cotton T-shirts to wear, which would be more comfortable, keep the jelly from getting on my clothes, and cause less disruption to the skin in the radiated area. Will I get through this treatment schedule just like thousands of other cancer patients before me? My answer is a resounding yes. I have no choice, and a positive attitude and gritted teeth can get you through a heck of a lot. Count me in on that game plan!

Some diminishment of how quickly my brain seems to be functioning is disconcerting. It is lovingly called "chemo brain." I call it annoying and frustrating. I sometimes make up new words from two different words. I'll call someone by the wrong name. I'll be talking along and just draw a blank on the subject matter or what to say next. I have found myself wanting to do my work as I normally would, but I have had to check and recheck to make certain I got everything right. I guess you will have to bear with me, and I ask for your forgiveness if I don't get something right. I keep being told that I should get better eventually, but the fatigue from the radiation treatments is compounding some of the brain function challenges following chemotherapy. I guess I am grateful for how well I have done to this point. Talk about being blessed!

Another concern has been the way the radiation treatments have affected my speaking and singing voice. Dr. Foster and I discussed that I have been having difficulty projecting when singing, and my voice has been hoarse at times. He did say that my vocal cords most likely are swollen because of the proximity to the radiation field, but this should be a short-term issue. Because I'm a vocalist, that was a relief to hear. I can only pray that God will give me back the full power of my voice when I successfully complete my treatments.

I will meet with a representative from clinical trials this morning to see if I am a candidate for the Metformin—a diabetes drug that has shown great promise in preventing the recurrence of breast cancer—clinical trial. I would take the drug twice per day for five years, in addition to the Tamoxifen, which has already been prescribed, and I will start taking it once I finish radiation treatments. It's lots to consider in terms of whether I want to sign on for an additional drug for five years, but I need to think about the elevated level of care being part of a clinical trial. I will find out more this morning and keep you in the loop.

So the journey continues to December 30. I got the not-so fun news that the radiation treatments will have a cumulative effect in the area being treated well into January of next year until I finally see some improvement. So although treatments end on December 30, I will have side effects for several more weeks. I ask that you continue offering prayers on my behalf that I will have enough strength, courage, and grit to get through these last treatments. Your support and prayers have carried me this far. We are almost across the finish line. Thank you! Love you.

Sunday, December 18, 2011, 11:42 a.m., CST

"You Can Do It"

Over the past week filled with daily radiation treatments, medical appointments, mailing presents, Christmas gatherings, work meetings, phone calls, processing year-end charitable gifts, preparing marketing and grant materials for the Impact-Cando Connection Fund, and taking my daily naps, I kept telling myself that I only had fourteen or thirteen or twelve or eleven or ten radiation treatments to go. I quite seriously would look in the mirror when tears filled my eyes and the pain would get intense and tell myself, "You can do it!" And I know I can. It is just getting there. I have tried not to think of what still lies ahead through the next nine treatments and the next four-plus weeks as my body tries to heal from this phase of my medical care.

The radiation oncology department has gone above and beyond to make certain I am comfortable:

- Recommending a new topical ointment for the radiated area

- Hugging me when I am smiling but overwhelmed with the process and my cheerful veneer starts to crack

- Arranging for me to see a massage therapist to get me to relax (like that is even possible)

- Coordinating my care with other departments so I can continue my journey back to health

- Consistently providing quality care, even on weekends, when I have had to ask the advice of an on-call radiation oncologist

I called Dr. Foster this morning when the skin on the fold under my left breast decided it wanted to open in areas and exposed some pretty raw skin and tissue underneath. Both Dr. Foster and I knew there might be an issue with this from the beginning. Simply put, when treating a breast cancer patient for the length of time required in my case in the area that is being treated on the low portion of the breast and I am a patient with significant breast tissue, it is a very real possibility that breakdown of the skin and tissue will occur, especially on the fold. So the inevitable has occurred, and I will work diligently to make certain I get through the rest of my treatments maintaining the radiated area as well as I can. Dr. Foster has reassured me that other prescribed ointments will help. Thank goodness! Yes, I know I can do it.

I did meet with Dr. Panwalkar, my phone nurse, and the clinical trials coordinator on Wednesday. I am happy to report that I have moved past the first section of getting enrolled in the Metformin clinical trial. My blood pressure was 122/77, I had lost 2.2 pounds in two days, and Dr. Panwalkar took me off three medications. So the next section of the workup for the clinical trial will be a twelve-hour fasting blood draw, a few other tests, and completion of associated questionnaires for the clinical trial study on the morning of December 28 following my radiation treatment that morning.

If I'm accepted into the clinical trial, it sounds as if I will start the Metformin for the first two weeks following completion of my radiation treatments on December 30, and then I will take Tamoxifen once it is known I have not had a reaction to the Metformin. Keep in mind that there is a fifty-fifty chance that I will be placed on a placebo rather than the Metformin as part of this clinical trial, but my medical team and I will not know what I am on because participants are assigned a number and then receive their medication from the pharmacy with the corresponding number. I will need to remember a few things when undergoing future scans that include coming off the Metformin drug two days prior to having a contrast dye administered to prevent kidney damage, as well as some B12 and other depletion, but blood tests will monitor those levels. All in all, the feedback from physicians who prescribe and patients who have been on Metformin has been positive, so we shall see what the future holds.

Jill and I will stay in Fargo for the Christmas and New Year's holidays, mostly because of my physical condition right now. Hopefully, it will be a quiet and relaxing time for us. Our mom will spend some time with us in Fargo over the next few weeks, too. Soon, I will regain my health and stamina and be able to more comfortably travel greater distances than around the Fargo area. As I mentioned in my last entry, sheer will, determination, grit, and patience will get me there. That and lots of prayers from all of you. Slowly but surely, I am reaching the end of my intense medical treatments, and I will graduate to the monitoring phase. Are we there yet?

As you start to gather for Christmas, I will offer up prayers that it is a peaceful, calm, and blessed time for you and your families. Enjoy and cherish each moment together. Thanks for keeping me in your prayers. Love you.

Tuesday, December 27, 2011, 6:45 p.m., CST

Down to Three

I am down to my last three radiation treatments, and the end of this phase is just in sight. The last two weeks have been very challenging in terms of caring for the radiation area. The skin continues to break down and will do so into the first few weeks of January, even though I finish my radiation treatments on December 30. The treatments have a cumulative effect on the area being treated, so I need to be very careful to avoid infection and stay in contact with Dr. Foster if things seem to change in terms of overall health of the radiation site.

I did visit with Dr. Foster this morning following my radiation treatment, and he has adjusted the size of the Mepilex silicone bandage covering being utilized on the radiation area. It is much larger, and he added a prescription cream, Silvadene, to help prevent and treat wound infections in patients with serious burns. Silver sulfadiazine stops the growth of bacteria that may infect an open wound. This decreases the risk of the bacteria spreading to surrounding skin or the blood, where it can cause a serious blood infection (sepsis). Silver sulfadiazine belongs to a class of drugs known as sulfa antibiotics.

Dr. Foster will see me again on Friday morning following my last treatment and again one week later to monitor the radiation area to make certain the skin and tissue are healing. It is a comfort knowing that he will watch me closely so I know things are going well. I have to say a big thank you to Nurse Jill Fuzzy Wuzzy, who has again been filling the role of one of my favorite children's book characters. She was the patient this morning for a root canal, so I will prompt her to take her pain medication on time so she is comfortable coming out of her procedure, too.

I begin a twelve-hour fast at 8:00 p.m. this evening for my blood work tomorrow morning to complete the second part of the Metformin clinical trial enrollment.

I also have been approved to take extra selenium and zinc to help with skin regeneration in the radiation area. A dear friend and internal medicine physician advised me to take these two supplements when I was going through my nose surgeries several years ago following skin cancer removal. They worked well then, and Dr. Foster indicated I could use them when I spoke with him this morning. He only requested that I wait until I finish my last treatment to start taking the supplements.

Jill, Mom, and I had a peaceful and relaxing three-day weekend for Christmas. We were able to talk via video conferencing to watch our family in the Twin Cities (Vicki, Tom, Betsy, Lissa, Logan, and Ally) open their Christmas presents, and they in turn got to watch us open ours. As much grief as we give Jill about all of her technology gadgets, we were happy we were able to be together, so to speak, on Christmas Eve and Day. We also had a chance to visit with Scott, Mark, Carla Ann, Ashley, Stephen, and a few aunts and uncles along the way. We are hoping to connect with a few others before New Year's.

So Friday, December 30, will soon be here, and the third phase of my treatments will be complete. For all of you who have so diligently traveled with me on my journey and kept me in your prayers, I will be forever grateful. 2012 will hopefully be a much better year for me, and I will embrace my new lease on life after successfully completing my breast cancer battle. After a few more steps, I will be there. Thanks for staying with me and praying for me as I complete this phase. My journey has forever changed me. Love you.

Friday, December 30, 2011, 12:20 p.m., CST

Phase III Completed

After thirty-three trips to the cancer center since November 14, I have finally completed the third phase of my breast cancer battle. I am thrilled and so looking forward to waking up each morning knowing that the challenging phases of my fight are over. It is hard to explain what normalcy means to a person who has been faced with a breast cancer diagnosis, but I will embrace my daily routine with everything I am and will smile ear to ear out of sheer joy for getting to do so.

I am still working to get enrolled in the Metformin clinical trial study, so I had to go through an abdominal ultrasound this morning to make certain I didn't have any issues with my liver. My blood work in that area was slightly out of range. So reassurances were necessary to move me forward with enrollment. I have placed my participation in this study in God's hands, so if I am accepted or not, I will be at peace with the decision. Either way, I will be on Tamoxifen for the next five years, and I will be monitored every three to four months over the same time period.

Nurse Jill Fuzzy Wuzzy continues to do a stellar job addressing some of my more than challenging breast skin and tissue breakdown areas. She has had to be brave as the caregiver just to apply various prescription salves and gels to the affected areas. I have appreciated her healing touch. Thank you, Jill! I love you for being there for me. My mom has been praying and worrying about getting me through the various stages of this battle since early April. Hey, Mom, we made it. I love you, too.

My family—Vicki and Tom, Betsy, Lissa (Logan and Ally), Mark and Carla Ann, Ashley, Stephen, Scott, and Kathy—have been lifting me up, picking up the pieces when things got dicey, and keeping the prayers coming. I love you for making me strong. Being from a large family, there are benefits, like having the tremendous support and prayers of my aunts and uncles, cousins, their spouses, and families through my whole journey. Thank you for being there for me. I love you all.

I cannot imagine how difficult this battle would have been without the support of my boss, all of my coworkers and their families, the board of directors, committee members and their families, former coworkers, business associates, my Cando connections, and many, many dear friends from quite literally all over the country. The prayer chains and all of your dedicated prayers and support have pulled me through my breast cancer fight. I am rejoicing today for your presence in my life. It is overwhelming and humbling. God truly has smiled on me, and I am thankful. I love you.

I am grateful for the tremendous care that the medical team at the Sanford Health's Roger Maris Cancer Center provided. When you think about the team members, who included Dr. Bouton and his nurses, Dr. Panwalkar and his nurses, my chemotherapy nurses (fourteen different ones), my radiation oncologists and their nurses, my PAs, radiation technologists (at least eight different ones), pharmacists, lab technicians, schedulers, receptionists, massage therapists, social workers, clergy, and greeters, my journey would not have been as successful and manageable without each and every one of them. They have guided me through a series of lifesaving treatments, side effects and all, and I have worked full time with the exception of a few weeks following my surgery. Thank you all for the wonderful care, compassion, love, hugs, and healing. When I completed my final radiation treatment, I was presented with a beautiful quilt that a volunteer to the radiation department donated. Pretty cool and incredibly thoughtful of someone to think of me with such a lovely remembrance. You have my love and gratitude.

Have I been blessed? More than I will ever know. Have I been forever changed? Definitely. I will never again take my life for granted and will continue to be thankful for my good fortune in being able to continue my life with a new, healthy outlook.

Thanks for traveling the long and winding path with me as I fought my way back to good health. I will never forget your compassion, kindness, support, and prayers. I have fought breast cancer, and I have won.

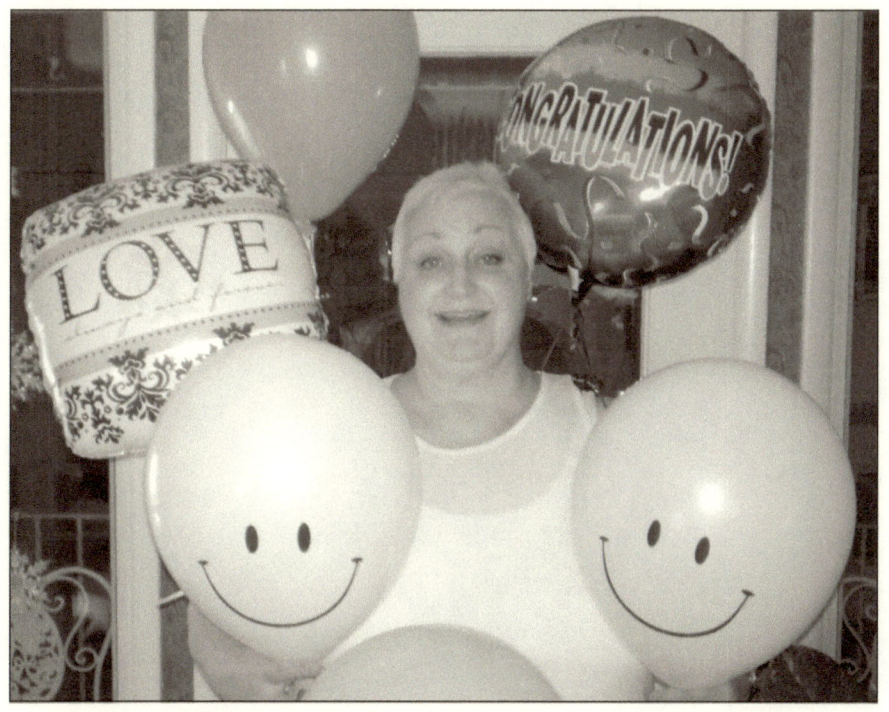

Mom and Jill wanted me to know how happy, proud, and relieved they were that I had made it through my formal breast cancer treatments, so they presented me with a bouquet of congratulatory balloons. Note the weary smile. I am finally done!

Have a wonderful 2012. I love you!

RECOVERY

Thursday, January 12, 2012, 7:28 a.m., CST

An Update on Healing

It has now been thirteen days since I finished my radiation treatments. The healing process has been challenging, and Nurse Jill continues to be at the ready to help with application of Silvadene, aloe gel, and bandages where needed. I see progress in the right direction, so I am thankful for the care and continued prayers. I will see Dr. Foster on January 20 so he can monitor the progress of the skin and tissue regrowth.

Fatigue, achy joints, lightheadedness, and difficulty with words and memory continue to be an issue, but with time, hopefully all of these will improve. I will need to keep working on my patience building, so I don't expect too much too soon.

I am happy to report that I was accepted on the Metformin clinical trial, and I am one of about eleven hundred in the United States and Canada who have been accepted into the study so far. My next appointment with Dr. Panwalkar is February 1. God willing, I will have a great checkup and be able to stay on course for a wonderfully fulfilling year.

I have met a number of people who are battling cancer in various forms, and gratefully, I have been able to share my experiences with surgery, chemo, and radiation to help them along in their battles. As personal as we all think this type of event should be, I can speak from experience in saying how grateful I have been for all people who have reached out to share their stories with me. By doing so, you alleviated fear, built confidence, and helped me avoid difficulties I would encounter on my journey. Thank you!

Recently, a woman who I met simply by being in the right place at the right time for less than five minutes reached out to me because she was awaiting a biopsy result, which came back positive for breast cancer. She had battled cervical cancer the previous fall, so it was, in my mind, God's hand that guided me to her desk and had us converse for less than five minutes about my breast cancer battle after she questioned me whether I was battling breast cancer. My pink, fuzzy cap and short, gray hair undoubtedly tipped her off.

Following our visit and her diagnosis of breast cancer the afternoon we spoke, she asked one of her coworkers, who knew me, to call me and ask me to call her so we could talk. She wanted to know what I was doing to stay so positive and to look so healthy as I fought through the various treatments. I was honored to call her the first night and several times since then to check in on her and see how things were going, and so far, she is doing well. When presented with opportunities to give back, you take them!

Thanks again for your support and prayers. Each day, I am getting a little better, and I have God and all of you to thank for that being the case. The saying that remains up in my room, "You never know how strong you are until being strong is the only choice you have," still is relevant today, not only for me, but the countless others who are battling cancer and other illnesses with the love of their families, friends, coworkers, medical team, and an army of many others we may never know who are praying for us. This type of event in your life brings out the very best in people and restores your faith in humanity. Life truly is good, and I am grateful I am still here to share in it. Love you.

Thursday, February 2, 2012, 7:58 a.m., CST

The Good News Continues

I had my three-month checkup with Dr. Panwalkar yesterday afternoon. He was very pleased with my progress. The skin and tissue have healed at the location where I had radiation treatments and my port removed, I have a full head of white hair, and I am making progress in terms of my overall strength and stamina. It will be six months to a year, most likely longer, before I gain back the ground I gave up to surgery, chemo, and radiation.

I will be more than happy to fight my way back because my prognosis is an excellent one. I know that my head/mind is getting stronger. It doesn't feel like I have a sense of vertigo as much anymore, and I take less pain medication each week. I still have moments of "blankness" or call someone by the wrong name and the occasional forgetfulness that accompanies chemo treatments. I just need to give myself time to recover. Quirky things like sores on my tongue, a tender left ankle, and painful right shoulder have cropped up, but hopefully, these too shall pass with care and time.

I am happy to be back on my nutritional products because they make me feel happier and healthier each day. Jill and I joined a women's gym, and we will start exercising in earnest now that I have approval to get back on my feet. I have been told to ease into a routine and not get too carried away. Slow and steady will win the race! I hope to get to the indoor golf facility this weekend to hit a few golf balls in preparation for our trip to South Carolina in early March. It has been nearly a year since I have swung a golf club or I have traveled out of the Fargo area due to my diagnosis and treatments. It is amazing what people take for granted every day, including me.

Today, I will start taking two Metformin tablets each day, along with the Tamoxifen prescription. So far, no major side effects have cropped up, so I am grateful.

Jill and I have been gearing up for the 2012 Giving Hearts Day event on February 14 because the Impact-Cando Connection Fund, for which we are fund advisors along with Rusty, has been selected to be a participant in this year's event. We have labeled and mailed hot pink postcards about the giving opportunity to the twenty-four hundred Cando alumni, worked with some key folks back in Cando to get the word out at home, and will continue to reach out leading up to the event through our website (www.candoconnection.org), Facebook, the local newspaper, e-mail, and personal contact.

We want folks aware that they can give back to the Cando area during the twenty-four hours of February 14 by giving a secure gift online through www.impactgiveback.org. Once you get to the website, click the Learn More button, then scroll down to the Impact-Cando Connection Fund, and click the Donate button next to our fund. From there, you can complete your gift of ten dollars or greater and even send an e-card if you so choose. Your gift will be doubled that day, thanks to our match sponsors who so graciously stepped up to participate. Thank you!

For those of you who know me well, you realize that this event has been a midrange goal for me to work toward as I was undergoing radiation treatments and recovery. It has been a positive event and will hopefully prove to be a successful and satisfying experience on February 14 for all people involved. I am grateful to be able to participate in the opportunity.

I continue to offer up prayers to the many people who I met through my journey who are also battling cancer. As I was reading a passage from a book yesterday, this part stuck with me throughout the day and sums up how I have felt over the last ten-plus months:

I have spread my wings of faith to embrace the "Wind," placing my heart in Jesus. I have experienced quiet, "everyday" miracles. His joy has balanced my pain, his power has lifted my burden, his peace has calmed my worries, his grace has been more than adequate to cover me, his strength has been sufficient to carry me through, and his love has bathed my wounds like a healing balm. Excerpt from "Why? Trusting God When You Don't Understand" by Anne Graham Lotz.

This passage sums up my feelings about how my breast cancer battle unfolded and my successful recovery to date. Through the blessings of God and all of your prayers and compassion, I am here to send a positive update. My next follow-up appointment is the end of March. My sincere thanks for continuing to offer up prayers, if you have some to spare, for my renewed health and a great 2012. Love you!

Wednesday, March 14, 2012, 6:30 a.m., CDT

Just a Few Challenges

I have received a number of e-mails inquiring how I am doing, so I am providing an update to bring you up to speed. I am now two and a half months past my formal treatments, and all in all, things seemed to be rolling along fairly well until I came down with a bad cold on February 1, which turned into a sinus and bronchial infection that I eventually needed to treat with an antibiotic. I can honestly say that God must have been riding my shoulder during my formal treatments because I did not contract the cold until a month after the end of my radiation treatments.

What you don't think about when going through breast cancer is that the area where your lymph nodes are removed (if necessary) and lumpectomies are completed can fill with fluid when you battle an infection. That weak area of your body cannot fight off the infection any more. I won't go into the details about how fun that part of the cold was. Suffice it to say, my body is working hard to reabsorb the fluid.

While battling the cold, I started experiencing severe muscle spasms in the hamstring areas on the back of both legs, making it difficult for me to walk, drive, and climb stairs and just generally undermining my confidence in walking or driving any great distances. The physicians and oncologists were not certain if the antibiotic were causing my symptoms, so my medication was switched to another to battle the sinus and bronchial infection.

I also made an appointment with a chiropractor who gave me three minor adjustments on my lower back. The last time I had been to his office was twenty-seven years ago, but I knew I had a bulged disc between the L4 and L5 area in my back, so I wanted to make certain a pinched nerve was not causing the leg spasms.

The leg spasms continued, so I was taken off Tamoxifen on February 21 and then Metformin on February 29. Both of these medications can cause some muscle issues. I was prescribed Valium as a muscle relaxer and used a capsaicin product on the affected areas. That made possible a trip to South Carolina with Jill that we had planned back in January to visit our family who live in that area. Dr. Panwalkar assured me that it was okay to travel, but I was to take my time and medications, relax, and, if possible, play some golf and get a hole in one. I could not ask for a more compassionate and caring medical oncologist. And Andrea, well, there are not enough nice words to describe how wonderfully she does her job and how supportive she has been.

Prior to leaving on the trip, I also had to work in my yearly physical with Dr. Ronald Wiisanen, who was his usual awesome self, highly encouraging and very thoughtful. He instructed me that, when I returned to Fargo, I was to fast for twelve hours for a blood draw to check a few things, including my TSH (thyroid levels). He also asked me to get a tetanus shot, but Dr. Wiisanen told me to wait until I got back so my arm would not be sore if I could golf. Bless his soul for thinking of that side effect.

So, Jill and I made the trip and had a wonderful time. We played golf six of the eight days we were there. I was able to complete five rounds of eighteen holes and one round of eleven holes. I recognized when I had to quit, and for most of you who know me, you know I don't do that easily. I had to concentrate very diligently in determining where to hit the golf ball close to the cart path and how I was going to walk up the various hills, onto the greens, and so forth because I was still experiencing some muscle spasms. The joy I felt in being able to connect with a golf ball made me cry and made me feel extremely grateful to God for letting me have the opportunity to play the game

I enjoy so much with my dear sister, Jill, who so lovingly cared for me through all of my treatments.

All of our relatives and friends made a concerted effort to get together or drove many miles to see Jill and me, and we were grateful to them for their thoughtfulness, hospitality, and encouragement to continue the good fight. We love you all for all you did and your special efforts to welcome us to South Carolina.

God saw fit to place me in some pretty incredible moments on this trip, where I could offer encouragement to others battling cancer or others who had completed their battle could share their stories with me to keep me positive and focused on the future. Whether on a plane or with friends, family, or folks in general, I was reminded that cancer is part of almost every person's life. I am getting God's message loud and strong that continuing to educate, offering encouragement, and being positive will now always be a part of my life.

Next on the medical agenda when I returned to Fargo was a trip to the dermatology department for a full body skin overview. I had skin cancer on my nose almost ten years ago now, and I have been asked to schedule an annual visit to monitor how things are going. That turned out fine. I will, however, need to have several other skin issues addressed in the next month or so and then, hopefully, will be good to go in that area for the time being.

It continues to amaze me the time and effort it takes to recover from going through this type of fight. Some days you feel great; other days, you feel highly fatigued. Managing stress is the key, so I am working to do that as well as I possibly can. I very much appreciate the understanding and compassion of the people who surround me on a daily basis. Thank you!

It also reminds me to never ever take anything for granted, to be grateful for every day I am on the face of the earth, and to make the most of each day. Within each of us are a fighting spirit and, hopefully, a recognition that we are not in total control of our lives. God is, and he will determine when, where, and how we will pass from this world. Until then, we need to accept the difficulties that we encounter in our lives with dignity, grace, and determination and know that he is constantly by our side.

To all of you who continue to keep me in your prayers and have been with me through this battle, thank you. I will persist in getting back on my feet, so to speak, and will work to be a healthier person so I can do the work that God has entrusted me to accomplish. Until I see you next, take care. Love you!

Thursday, March 22, 2012, 12:50 p.m., CDT

Providing an Update

I honestly thought that, when I completed my chemo and radiation treatments, I would be good to go, so to speak, health wise. I thought I would just need to start taking the prescribed cancer-fighting drug and clinical trial drug and everything would move along smoothly. I would be back at the gym on the treadmill, lifting some light weights, getting ready to walk my eighteen holes of golf with Jill each Saturday and Sunday morning, and preparing for the 5K race as part of the local marathon. Well, not so fast there, "Feeling Older on the Inside and Outside" Lady!

The severe muscle spasms in the hamstring areas on the back of both legs and now incredibly achy knees continue to make it difficult for me to walk, drive, climb stairs, and be active. (Boy, do I have a much greater appreciation of what my mother and brother-in-law are going through.) I kept thinking it was because of the tetanus shot I had on March 14, but after visiting with Dr. Panwalkar on March 19, we think it is more likely a combination of a number of things—chemo drugs still in my system, the cancer-fighting drugs I was taking, general fatigue from making my trip to South Carolina, and, yes, my thyroid level being out of range.

That is right. Last Thursday morning, March 15, I was informed that my twelve-hour fasting TSH level blood work had come back at 10.8. The last time I had my thyroid level checked was back in October 2011, between chemo and radiation treatments, and it was 1.4. The normal range is 0.4 to 5.1, so my thyroid medication dosage has been increased and will be monitored to see if it comes down. The additional concern is that I have a nodule on the left side of my thyroid that has had two needle biopsies in the past five years, monitoring for potential cancer. There is some concern that, with all of the radiation on my left side and near the lymph nodes right next to the thyroid, there may be an issue with the thyroid.

I was asked to get additional thyroid-related blood work done today, March 22, and I will have an ultrasound of the thyroid on March 28, followed by an appointment with Dr. Julie Hallanger-Johnson, my endocrinologist, on the morning of March 29. I am praying for good news and that the thyroid level will eventually return to a normal range. The higher thyroid reading could explain the muscle spasms in my legs, achy knees, hair loss, chills, and weight gain I have been experiencing. So hopefully, the additional thyroid medication can help that issue, God willing. One step at a time! I am hanging in there and trying to stay positive.

During the March 19 appointment with Dr. Panwalkar, he took me off the Valium and capsaicin product and prescribed Metaxalone (eight hundred milligrams) twice per day in the hopes I would finally start to regain some normalcy in the hamstrings and knees. There has been a slight improvement, so as of this morning, he put me back on Metformin (once per day) to see how I tolerate that medication.

I am still off the Tamoxifen, and we will do an additional blood test to see what other drug options might be available to me once we know I can tolerate the Metformin and once my thyroid level starts to move closer to being in range.

As you might recall, I didn't really slow down much during my chemo and radiation treatments, so I think God is sending me a message to slow down a bit now by throwing a few curveballs at me when I think I should be back to my normal self. I can only continue to put one foot in front of the other, manage my stress level, stay positive, and offer up my fight to God, asking that he sees fit to eventually return me to a healthier state.

If you wonder if I get frustrated and cry because I want to be achieving my short- and long-term goals, the answer is yes. Do I continue to pout and feel sorry for myself for too long? The answer is no. I have my mom, siblings, other family members, my boss, coworkers, and many, many friends who won't let me mope for too long. Thank you all for staying the course with me in prayer and support. I will keep fighting and keep you informed as things proceed. I know God is with me in my battle.

On a positive note, I received a call last Friday from Radiation Oncology, inviting me to be a featured speaker at their upcoming open house unveiling some of the new facilities they have completed at the cancer center. I guess my name was the first one that came up because it was felt I had been an inspiration to other patients and the staff while I was undergoing radiation treatments. Their recognition and request humbled me, but I graciously declined the offer because I felt I was not in a good place health wise just yet to be a worthy spokesperson. Just know I try to help others battling cancer and illnesses in different ways as often as I can because so many of you have been an inspiration to me as I walked the path of my breast cancer battle.

The journey continues, and hopefully, in my next update, I will be able to provide more positive news about how things are going. For all of you who continue to offer up prayers, support, and encouragement, my sincere thanks! Until I see you next, take care. Love you!

Friday, March 30, 2012, 7:30 a.m., CDT

Additional News

I had mixed news yesterday. My thyroid level is moving back toward a more normal level thanks to my new medication, but a new nodule has appeared on the left side of my thyroid. Dr. Hallanger-Johnson will need to do a needle biopsy on that nodule on April 19 to see if it is cancerous. She also suspects that I may have developed a form of arthritis, especially in my knees, as a side effect of my breast cancer battle and all the different types of drugs, so I have additional blood work this morning to see if that is the case.

I am still experiencing severe achiness, down to my bones over most of my body, and muscle spasms in the hamstring area on the backs of my legs, even while taking medications to try to address these issues. Dr. Hallanger-Johnson and Dr. Panwalkar have both reassured me that we will continue to work toward a solution. All of the chemo drugs, steroids, radiation, and now cancer-fighting drugs can really throw the thyroid hormones out of whack, so I know they will work together to make good decisions for me long term.

I already had been diagnosed with Hashimoto's disease, an autoimmune disease that continually attacks the thyroid gland, a number of years ago, but I had been able to control the thyroid level through taking a thyroid medication every morning. I have a larger nodule also on the left side of my thyroid that has reduced slightly in size. Two needle biopsies had been done on that nodule in the past five years, so when I heard a new area was revealed during my ultrasound procedure yesterday morning, it was unsettling. I will once again ask God to help get me through whatever lies ahead.

Dr. Hallanger-Johnson asked if I were feeling any differently because my one-year anniversary of being diagnosed with breast cancer (April

12) was coming up. I laughed because one of my coworkers recently mentioned something about celebrating on April 12, and I asked her what was important about that date. So my answer to Dr. Hallanger-Johnson was that I quite simply just want to be back on my feet, being somewhat active and not in as much pain. I am more frustrated than anything, not depressed, but I also resolved to regain some of the ground that I have lost.

On another note, Dr. Hallanger-Johnson also told me that, because of the Hashimoto's disease, I needed to bring down my stress levels and give my body time to heal because stress is one of the greatest triggers that bring on issues with the thyroid. She said she was joining the chorus along with the rest of my physicians, nurses, and technicians about shortening my workday, and that meant at home, too, giving my body time to recover from what it has just been through over the past year.

So I will continue to do what I can to address that issue. Thanks for your understanding if I don't just jump to getting something done or if you don't hear back from me right away. It will be difficult for me to make this type of adjustment because being busy has always been the way I have lived my life. But a change is necessary, and I will make it for my own health and hopefully longevity of life.

My first official mammogram and follow-up after that scan with Dr. Bouton is scheduled for April 12. That date is merely a coincidence because it was originally scheduled for April 13 and his schedule changed, so it had to be rescheduled. And that happened to be the date that was selected. As I find out more information on all of the tests, I will keep you informed.

Meanwhile, if you would, please continue to keep me in your prayers that I will have good news following the upcoming mammogram and needle biopsy on my thyroid. Your support and prayers have carried me through so much already. I almost feel guilty in asking, but I do know the power of prayer so that is why I ask you to continue sending them my way. I continue to offer up my journey to God and will walk the path to wherever it may lead. Until I see you next, take care! Love you!

Friday, April 20, 2012 7:44 a.m., CDT

Standing Firm

> *When I don't understand why, I trust him because God is always on time for his purposes in my life.* Excerpt from "Streams in the Desert" by L.B. Cowman.

Since the last time I updated my journal, I have received answers to some of our prayers, and I am still awaiting final test results on others. After undergoing blood tests for rheumatoid arthritis and lupus, I am happy to report that both of those blood tests came back within a normal range. Thank you, God! I am still battling very painful joints, especially in my knees, so I have added a joint support supplement with glucosamine, extra selenium, copper, and manganese to the supplements I take each day, and it has started to help take away some of the pain. Yesterday, I was asked to increase my dosage of Metformin to two pills per day, so I made the transition in the afternoon.

The muscle spasms in my hamstrings continue to be an issue, so I still take two Metaxalone pills per day to keep me up and moving as well as I can. I hope that, as soon as my thyroid level gets into the normal range (0.40–5.00), the muscle spasms will improve. The reading from blood work completed on Tuesday of this week shows I am currently at 6.38, still outside of range.

My first official mammogram and follow-up after that scan with Dr. Bouton was on April 12, my first-year anniversary. The mammogram revealed what it always had, no potential breast cancer issues. However, I had mentioned to Dr. Panwalkar several weeks ago and also Dr. Bouton during our appointment that I had been having some eerily familiar breast pain in three spots on my left breast, away from the areas that had been radiated and where Dr. Bouton performed the double lumpectomy and lymph node removal. With that information in mind and to make certain we were diligent in not overlooking a potential medical issue, I underwent an ultrasound procedure yesterday morning (April 19) on the three sore areas.

The appointment had a déjà vu type of feeling to it. The medical team indicated it was still very difficult to read the mammogram because of the density of my breast tissue, and the radiologist came into the room to ask the technicians to rescan the areas of concern, based on their initial scans. Essentially, he did not feel the sore spots were areas of concern, other than normal pain associated with my breast cancer battle, and no further tests have been ordered at this time. So, chalk up a victory for my one-year breast cancer anniversary. My heart was much lighter, and I thanked God for that good news.

Dr. Hallanger-Johnson performed a needle biopsy on a new nodule on the left side of my thyroid yesterday afternoon (April 19) to see if it is cancerous. Initially, I was told I would only have to endure two needles being inserted for the biopsy, so after four needles, with only some topical cream applied to my neck to help with deadening the area, I was glad to be done.

A bubble of blood appeared after the first needle was inserted, which was held pressure to, but I am bruised, the area is swollen this morning, and it hurts to talk and swallow. I will call to see what we can do to help manage the pain today. The test results will take several days to come back, so I will update you as soon as I know the results. Thanks, Jill, for being by my side for this procedure. Your presence and sense of humor were a blessing.

After the biopsy was completed, Dr. Hallanger-Johnson and I discussed the merits of increasing my thyroid medication dosage to eventually get me back into a normal range. Hopefully, this will eventually help me with the muscle spasms in the hamstring area on the backs of my legs, as well as my fatigue, hair loss, chills, weight gain, and dry skin.

Dr. Hallanger-Johnson and Dr. Panwalkar are working together so, when I start taking my new breast cancer-fighting drug, Anastrozole (one milligram), once per day, my thyroid levels will stay in range. I will start that medication once we hear back on the thyroid biopsy results. God willing, I hope the results bring good news.

Dr. Hallanger-Johnson talked with me again yesterday about how important it was for me to bring down my stress levels, especially with my Hashimoto's disease diagnosis, and to give my body time to heal because stress is one of the greatest triggers that bring on thyroid issues. I was happy to report to her that I had been making a concerted effort to shorten my days and get more rest, ultimately giving my body time to recover from what it had been through over the past year.

For those of you who have offered a helping hand at work or elsewhere, thank you! Thanks for understanding that it will be difficult for me to make this type of adjustment because being busy has always been the way I have lived my life. The saying "All in good time" seems appropriate here. I will continue to rest and relax more for my own good health.

A friend undergoing breast cancer treatments left a voice message for me on Monday, and when I called her back, she wanted to know if I had lost any fingernails or toenails, whether I had tingling in my hands and feet, toes, and fingers or on my tongue and around the mouth, or if I had swollen ankles and feet while undergoing chemo. She also indicated she has had two blood transfusions (a total of four units) during her chemo treatments. After we compared notes, I thanked her for the call because I oftentimes thought I was the patient with the odd symptoms and she made me feel more normal.

She also made me feel blessed, not only because she confirmed that I truly was fortunate during my breast cancer treatments not to have life-threatening side effects, but also because she felt comfortable enough to call me as a mentor, so to speak. I reassured her that she sounded great and to hang in there. I knew she would make it, and I was praying for her. Just as so many of you have done for me over the past year once you knew of my diagnosis, thank you!

A dear friend of mine, a former Candoite, made a special trip to our condo on my one-year anniversary on April 12 with his ice cream truck. Thank you, Pat, for your thoughtfulness, generosity, and prayers. Pretty cool to be remembered in such a special way, not only for me but for Jill, my primary caregiver, too. No doubt, the neighborhood kids were also glad to see you.

To those of you who continue to keep me in your prayers, thank you so much. Your support and prayers have been so encouraging to my family and me during this challenging journey. I can only pray that I will continue to get good news as I continue down my path to renewed health and can help others who may be diagnosed with a cancerous situation.

Finally, my Bible verse yesterday included these words, which I was obviously meant to read prior to my two procedures:

Stand firm and you will see the deliverance the Lord will bring you today (Ex. 14:13).

Even in the worst of times, God would have me be cheerful and courageous, rejoicing in His love and faithfulness.

And if for a season He calls me to "stand firm," I will acknowledge it as time to renew my strength for greater strides in the future. Excerpt from "Streams in the Desert" by L.B. Cowman.

Until I see you next, take care! Love you!

Friday, May 4, 2012 7:32 a.m., CDT

Just Simply Being Grateful

Faith, when walking through the dark with God, only asks Him to hold his hand more tightly. Excerpt from "Streams in the Desert" by L.B. Cowman.

The medical issues continue to occur, and I am taking it one day at a time, sometimes one hour at a time. Since completing my formal treatments on December 30, 2011, I have had to have:

- A follow-up ultrasound to confirm that my left breast tissue was normal (and it does remain cancer free)

- A thyroid biopsy to make certain a new nodule was not cancerous (which came back as normal)

- A cyst removed from my back (which was also found to be benign)

- Multiple blood and other tests (which confirmed that my thyroid level is still out of range compared to where it has been the past ten years)

I currently take a higher dose of thyroid medication to address the situation. Ironically enough, I have recently spoken to several people also having thyroid issues, and hopefully sharing knowledge has helped alleviate some of their concerns. God does work in mysterious ways. I still experience tremendous muscle spasms at times and achy knees, ankles, feet, shoulders, and hands most of the time. I pray each day that God will grant me the patience to cope and long-term health.

Last Friday afternoon, I was diagnosed with a urinary tract infection, which I have not had for nearly twenty years. I have had allergic reactions to some of my prescribed medications, including the one recently prescribed for the urinary tract infection, which is always scary. Thankfully, Benadryl to counteract the allergic reaction and a new medication helped to clear the infection, and I am finally starting to feel better.

I have remained on the Metformin clinical trial drug for nearly two months; however, the breast cancer-fighting medication has been challenging. I am off Tamoxifen, and my Anastrozole prescription has been suspended until my thyroid is back in range, at least until June 15. The side effects were more than I could handle for the time being, and the people who truly know me understand that I don't give up easily.

I never know what will happen each day, so I just place my trust in God and put one foot in front of the other and keep going. My prognosis is still excellent. It is just getting by all of the side effects of the rigorous treatments I endured last year and the fallout from the heavy-duty drugs that were prescribed. If I had not been diagnosed with the most aggressive form of breast cancer, I might choose not to take the drugs being prescribed. But I don't have that choice if I want to do what is best for my long-term health.

With the various breast cancer-fighting medications and the tremendous side effects of the chemo and radiation treatments I endured, my doctors have indicated that my body is still trying to heal and issues may crop up as far out as four years from now.

They are reassuring me that, eventually, over the next five years or so, I will start to feel a bit more like normal. I have a new appreciation of the times in the past I asked someone who had battled cancer how she was doing, and a wry smile crossed her face before she updated me on her health status. It makes sense now.

I have found that the best medicine is a smile on my face, adequate rest, and maintaining a positive attitude. Embracing all of those things will certainly help me jump any hurdles that are thrown up as I continue my journey. You just never know what lies ahead, and I mean that sincerely. I and everyone else I know should rejoice in the wonderfully resilient bodies we have been blessed with, and we also need to thank God for our health, in whatever shape it is in each day, because things could be much worse.

Had I not seen my brother succumb to brain cancer at the age of twenty-one after a four-year battle, I know I would not be as strong as I have been and continue to be today. Our family and friends learned very valuable lessons through his experience, and I have tried, along with my family, to approach my cancerous situation in a different manner. Perhaps more lightheartedly and with a sense of humor, it is all a matter of perspective and determination when you hear the words, "You have cancer." You just fight with everything you have and all you are. Simply being able to heal and continuing my life is priceless.

If I have learned nothing else, it is to trust in God to guide my future and to continue to have patience for the long term—patience to know I should allow myself the time to recover, patience when my body is just not cooperating, and patience to know that God knows best what I can endure in his name.

So, the healing continues. The most important thing that you can do is continue to offer up prayers for my long-term health and healing. Just know I am grateful for your support, compassion, and prayers. It has been a long journey so far.

Faith is recognizing God's promise as an actual fact, believing it is true, rejoicing in the knowledge of that truth, and then simply resting because God said it. Excerpt from "Streams in the Desert" by L.B. Cowman.

Love you.

Tuesday, May 22, 2012, 7:58 a.m., CDT

Another Year Older

And, hopefully, much wiser! Today, I am so blessed to be turning fifty-four years old. When I was first diagnosed with breast cancer, a part of me did not know if I would live to see this day. I am so grateful that I have made it. A recent spiritual passage I read has stayed with me:

> *The pressure of difficult times makes us value life. Every time our life is spared and given back to us after a trial, it is like a new beginning. We better understand its value and thereby apply ourselves more effectively for God and for humankind. And the pressure we endure helps us to understand the trials of others, equipping us to help them and to sympathize with them.* Excerpt from "Streams in the Desert" by L.B. Cowman.

I recently received a call from a woman who is just completing chemo and beginning her radiation treatments in the next week or so for breast cancer. She had questions regarding side effects and wanted to know if I were affected in a similar manner and what I did to cope. I just opened up and shared with her because God would want me to do that, to try to lift up another going through a difficult health ordeal. He has uniquely equipped me with the knowledge and understanding as to:

- Why we have days that are highs and days that are lows

- Why he brings us to the brink of what we think we can handle and why he pulls us back into safety and peace

- Why he spares us so we can reach out and help others placed in similar circumstances

One never knows from day to day when her time will come to leave the face of this earth. You live by faith, love, hope, and charity, trying to make the best decisions possible in your life. In my case, I also pray that God will spare me further pain and place his hand upon me with healing and a renewed sense of well-being—physical, emotional, and spiritual. Slowly but surely, my prayers are being answered.

Another area of concern has cropped up and I have an appointment this Thursday for an oral surgeon to look more closely at a spot on my tongue. The area, right in the middle of my tongue, has been changing color and texture and growing in size over the past several months. Having been diagnosed with cancer twice in my life, I do not take anything looking unusual for granted anymore. I have vowed to be proactive rather than reactive. I did visit with my dentist prior to making this new appointment, and we have tried to address the area of concern with Nystatin, with me swishing and swallowing the medication four times per day, but I have not yet seen improvement in the area. So I will keep my appointment to see the oral surgeon, once again erring on the side of caution. I am praying for a good appointment.

I also decided a week ago, Monday, May 14, to stop the Metformin clinical trial drug for the time being. I have not yet recovered from the muscle spasms, joint pain, lightheadedness, bloating, and generally feeling achy all over. In the week or so since suspending the Metformin, I have felt just a little stronger and more stable. Every morning that I swing my legs over the side of the bed, I pray that, when I stand up, I will feel more like my old self. I keep hoping I don't have to accept that my body has a new normal feeling, one that I don't really like, but I have come to accept as part of what I will be feeling while my body continues to heal from all it endured in the last thirteen-plus months.

I try to keep a smile firmly on my face because I have so much to be thankful for in my life. And today, more than any other day during the year, I will celebrate that I am alive and, for the most part, doing well. So many don't get the prognosis I received. That just simply makes my heart hurt. I pray each and every day that God will have mercy on those who have not received a positive prognosis and he will hold them in his hands as they approach the end of their lives. And I pray for a cure for cancer. What a wonderful thing that would be!

So today, I rejoice in knowing my life stretches positively in front of me. I thank God for the tremendous family, friends, boss, coworkers, board and committee members, survivors, support team in Cando or wherever you are, and the wonderful medical team who have carried me through the past one-plus year of my breast cancer battle and all that entails. I have been blessed beyond measure, and I am grateful.

As Jill wrote in her birthday card message, "Let's try to make it another year, okay?" You can count on me giving 100 percent to make that wish come true! Just know how much I love everyone for his or her continued prayers, thoughts, and well-wishes. Love you!

Sunday, June 3, 2012, 8:45 a.m., CDT

Knowing When to Ask for Help

I received good news during my appointment with the oral surgeon regarding my tongue. I have a condition called medial rhomboid glassitis, or balding of the tongue. This condition can happen to anyone, and the oral surgeon has indicated it is most likely a permanent condition. However, he also indicated he felt it was not a cancerous situation. So once again, God has smiled on me.

Jill and I made it back to Cando, and for me, it was the first time I was back in my hometown in over one and a half years. It was nice to see Mom at our family home and to sleep in my childhood room. It was also comforting to help plant the cemetery where my dad, brother, grandparents, aunts, uncles, and numerous friends are buried. It has become a bit of a tradition for Jill, Mom, and me to plant the cemetery. We missed it last year while I was recovering from my breast cancer surgery.

We saw so many people from Cando who were there to plant or place flowers for their loved ones. Many have been right by my side through this whole ordeal. It was a joy to hug them, greet them with a smile, and thank them for the prayers, cards, e-mails, and just plainly being there.

When we arrived in Cando on Friday evening, I was not feeling well following the long ride, and it took some rest and care by my trusted caregivers to get me back to feeling better that evening. For the following days, it rained quite a bit, so we enjoyed our time together indoors, tackling small repairs, cooking and visiting. Nothing too stressful. Just time well spent!

Following our trip back to Fargo, I awoke Tuesday morning feeling incredibly lethargic. I had no energy. So I rested and slept most of the day Tuesday and went to sleep with a headache. I awoke Wednesday morning, still bothered by a headache, and finally pulled out my blood pressure cuff to check to see if it were part of the problem. When my blood pressure read 174/114, Dr. Panwalkar asked me to go to the walk-in clinic.

I drove myself. My former family medicine physician saw me, and following some tests, I was told I was most likely battling a viral infection and I needed to go home to rest and try to get my blood pressure down.

I left the walk-in clinic, sat in my car to make four phone calls to Mom, Jill, Pat (my boss), and the office to let them know I would not be in and was asked to go home and rest. I did not want to drive and make phone calls at the same time. I wasn't feeling that well and thought it would be safer just to stay put to make the calls. I then sat in the sunshine for about five minutes because we had not seen much of that for the few days prior and just soaked up the sun.

I took a deep breath, put my car in reverse, and looked in my rearview mirror, which has backup assist. I saw nothing, so I started to back up and then hit a vehicle driving quickly through the patient parking lot. It wasn't really what I needed to have happen when my blood pressure was so high. The rest of that time is a bit of a blur for me. I know I talked with the two men in the van that I hit, my insurance company, and a Fargo policewoman, who wrote up the accident.

I did manage to make it back to the condo and then finally shared with Mom and Jill that I had been living through some extraordinary pain in my left breast for the past five months following radiation. Every time I battle an infection, the breast tissue retains fluid because the lymph nodes in that area have been removed. A large share of the tissue in that breast that was radiated is hard as well.

I had mentioned the painful condition to my doctors, and if you recall, an ultrasound of the breast was done earlier this spring, and no further cancerous condition was found. Don't get me wrong. I was so very grateful there was nothing more to be concerned about in terms of cancer. However, the constant pain and, at times, more excruciating pain, have finally taken a toll.

I reached out to my friend, Joanne, at the cancer center on Thursday morning. I basically told her I could not handle the pain any longer. I told her that I had pasted a smile on my face, tried to have a positive attitude, and just tried to be brave in the hopes the pain would dissipate over the last few months. It has not, and Dr. Panwalkar confirmed that on Friday at 3:45 p.m. when I saw him and he did an exam.

He had barely started to examine the area when he hit a very sore spot and I flinched. He jumped back, looking at me rather stunned. I think for the first time that he understood what I had been going through and what I had not truly shared with other people. He told me he was going to visit with Dr. Foster and he would be back. I sat there and waited, praying I would finally get some help with the pain.

When he returned, he indicated he would be prescribing a cream that had to be specially mixed, which contains 4 percent Amitriptyline, 10 percent Ketamine, and 10 percent Lidocaine. We had talked about oral medications, but I did not want to become dependent on oxycodone or Valium, two of the pain medications I had used during my breast cancer battle. So I picked up the cream late Friday afternoon, and I have been using it three times per day to try to cope better with the intense pain that has been a part of my life since finishing my radiation treatments on December 30. It has been a challenge over the past five months to try to stay ahead of the pain, using ibuprofen and other coping skills, but I finally could not handle it any longer and knew I needed to ask for help.

For all of us, there is a need to be strong and resilient and to reassure our loved ones and those folks who have been with us on our walks that everything will be okay. If you know me at all, you know I hate to admit defeat, but I finally did what I think was right for me, ask for help. In the time ahead, I may not always have a smile on my face or seem upbeat and positive. Just know I am trying to fight my way back. Evidently, the breast pain is something that will be with me for quite some time. It is inherent to all I have endured over the past year in battling down breast cancer. My respect and admiration for those who have walked in these shoes continues to grow. God bless you for your strength and resolve and also for reaching out to help others along the way.

My Bible reading yesterday said:

If you are enduring great afflictions right now, you are at the source of the strongest faith. God will touch you during these dark hours to have the most powerful bond to His throne you could ever know, if you will only submit. Don't be afraid, just believe. But if you are afraid, just simply look up and say, "When I am afraid, I will trust in you." Then you will be able to thank God for his school of sorrow that became for you the school of faith. Great faith must first endure great trials. God's greatest gifts come through great pain. Excerpt from "Streams in the Desert" by L.B. Cowman.

Undoubtedly, God is sending me a message to stay strong and endure and to trust in him. As I have done all along through this journey, I will continue to offer this walk up to God.

I give my most sincere thanks for walking and praying with me through my battle. I take comfort in knowing you are all there, as is God. Love you.

Saturday, June 30, 2012, 3:50 p.m., CDT

With Patience I Wait

I wait for the restoration of a more normal life, one with less pain, aches, confusion, uncertainty, and worry. I read this spiritual passage the other day, which calmed some of my fears and gave me renewed hope:

> *No, my friend, it is not raining afflictions on you. It is raining tenderness, love, compassion, patience, and a thousand other flowers and fruits of the blessed Holy Spirit. And they are bringing to your life spiritual enrichment that all the prosperity and ease of this world could never produce in your innermost being.* Excerpt from "Streams in the Desert" by L.B. Cowman.

Some of my medical issues have been resolved; others are being addressed but will obviously take more time. My latest thyroid test came back two weeks ago, and I am finally back in range. With that good news came another attempt to get me back on Tamoxifen. I was only able to take it two days before my muscles became so rigid that I could barely walk and function. Once again, Dr. Panwalkar told me to stop taking the medication until my body had more time to heal. So with patience, I wait for the next opportunity to take medication that may help prevent the recurrence of my breast cancer.

After thinking through some of my symptoms and side effects like my balding tongue issue, continuing muscle spasms, lightheadedness, balance issues, and numbness in my hands, feet, lips, and tongue, I recently pieced together that I might have a B12 vitamin deficiency. I was on and off Metformin during a clinical trial over a period of time since January of this year, and I had read and been told that it might cause depletion of B12. Additionally, having Hashimoto's disease, I could also be at a higher risk of developing a B12 deficiency. The oral surgeon I saw to diagnose my tongue issue said during his exam that this condition might stem from a lack of vitamins.

Following discussion with the walk-in physician I saw about ten days ago, I have increased my intake of B12 and seen some improvement on my tongue and my general overall well-being. I was told it would take between three to four weeks to see any major improvement, so once again, with patience, I wait.

The cream I mentioned in my last journal entry and e-mail has helped take the edge off my breast pain. But it is still there every day. The use of the cream has just minimized it.

One of the timeliest bits of information I received recently was a newsletter article that the cancer center issued about peripheral neuropathy, which was hugely informative for me and, no doubt, countless others. Some of the highlights, which relate directly to my experiences, indicated that cancer treatment side effects are wide-ranging and can be long lasting. If you've ever felt numbness, pain, or burning sensations in your hands, feet, or legs, you may have experienced what physicians refer to as peripheral neuropathy, a condition that affects many cancer patients both during and after the duration of their cancer therapy.

The article said that the body is made up of complex neurological pathways that send signals from the brain to other parts of the body so we know where our body exists in space. Some of these pathways and nerves outside of the brain (central nervous system) are the peripheral nervous system.

Symptoms of peripheral neuropathy are wide-ranging and can affect motor, sensory, and autonomic nerves. When the sensory nerves are affected, you can feel pain, tingling, or numbness. When the motor nerves are affected, you may feel cramps, twinges, weakness, and even loss of muscle bulk. When the autonomic system, which regulates the automatic occurrences in the body such as blood pressure and sweating, is affected, you may experience excessive sweating, diarrhea, orthostatic hypertension, and so forth. With neuropathy, some patients even describe not being able to tell where their bodies or limbs are in space when they close their eyes or walk in a dark room.

Additional information in the article addressed causes of peripheral neuropathy, including vitamin deficiencies, kidney disease, hypothyroidism, autoimmune disorders, and certain anti-cancer medications, among other causes. When cancer treatment is the culprit, it may be due to the type of cancer or the type of treatment prescribed. In my case, treatment included several of the drugs listed. In fact, depending on the type of chemotherapy you get, up to 40 percent of patients experience some form of peripheral neuropathy. Two-thirds of these patients have symptoms lasting six months or longer. In some cases, the neuropathy worsens before it gets better following treatment.

I am happy to report that, over the course of my chemo treatments and in the months following, Dr. Panwalkar has worked to try to alleviate my issues via gabapentin (Neurontin), capsaicin, and, most recently, the specially mixed prescription cream that includes drugs listed in the informative article.

Essentially, I realized after reading the article that a number of the medical issues I have been experiencing are directly related to the chemo I underwent to beat my breast cancer as well as several other medical conditions I have had for a number of years, which my rigorous chemo treatments no doubt exacerbated.

At times, I've questioned my sanity, why I don't feel comfortable driving at night or long distances, why I feel so fatigued, why I hurt all over and then have specific areas with sharp, excruciating pain, why I almost fall over at times when I stand up and am lightheaded at other times, and why I know my blood pressure is out of control at times and then perfectly fine at others. It has been a roller coaster of emotions and a huge challenge physically to find some solid ground. The few times I find it, I am so grateful to feel a sense of normalcy that I find myself laughing almost hysterically because I have finally found some peace and calm, away from fear and worry.

I finally saw a psychologist at the cancer center about two weeks ago, who encouraged me to find more time to rest and relax and truly give my body and mind a chance to heal following this long, drawn-out medical ordeal. She made me face several facts that I was trying to avoid and told me it was normal to have anxiety and fear and to worry about what was lying ahead. My feelings were normal and expected. In essence, she told me to give myself a break from wearing the brave and cheerful mask I have worn for the past one-plus years. I think my shoulder and neck muscles relaxed following that appointment for the first time since I was diagnosed with breast cancer, and it felt good.

So with patience, I wait to feel better, to get a chance to play some much anticipated golf, and to wake each morning with less aches, pain, and worry. But I do so knowing that I have so much more to be grateful for because I am here and, all in all, doing well. When I need something positive to focus on, I remember my prognosis and the hundreds of people who have walked this path with me, rocks, stumbles, and all. Your generosity of spirit continues to amaze me; your compassion and prayers humble me. "Thank you" seems so inadequate. Just know I say it from my heart, which is where you and God continue to reside. My final thoughts are once again from a recent spiritual reading:

When conflict comes and the battle rages on, they become discouraged and surrender. Difficult times and places are our schools of faith and character. If we are ever to rise above mere human strength, and experience the power of the life of Christ in our mortal bodies, it will be through the process of conflict. Dear child of God, you may be suffering, but you cannot fail if you will only dare to believe, stand firm, and refuse to be overcome. Excerpt from "Streams in the Desert" by L.B. Cowman.

Love you.

Saturday, August 4, 2012, 8:10 a.m., CDT

The Calm and Then the Storm

If we would look at our past, most of us would realize that the times we endured the greatest stress and felt that every path was blocked were the very times our heavenly Father chose to do the kindest things for us and bestow his richest blessings. Excerpt from "Streams in the Desert" by L.B. Cowman.

Since my last journal entry/e-mail, my life truly has been like the calm before the storm. When I look back on my recent calendar, the week of the Fourth of July had no medical appointments noted. Can that possibly be right? No wonder I was feeling so calm and peaceful on the inside at that time. The only thing noted, outside of work, was an appointment for a pedicure, an indulgence I relish even more now because, during my formal treatments, I wasn't able to have my toenails polished with any color. Now my favorite polish color is anything in pink.

Coming out of the Fourth of July weekend, I had pain from a tooth my dentist and I had intended to crown about one and a half years ago, but we were prevented from fixing because of my breast cancer battle. So with the painful area starting to abscess, I endured a root canal on July 12, following several other dental visits to make certain we were on the right course of action. Suffice it to say, I will chew on the right side of my mouth for some time into the future until a permanent crown is put in place.

The week of July 16 started with a three-month follow-up appointment with Dr. Panwalkar, and we talked about:

- Some of the overall aches and pains I had been continuing to feel

- The importance of trying to lose some of the weight I had gained (which would definitely help my long-term recovery)

- My ongoing breast pain

The pain is primarily in the left breast due to the extensive scar tissue from radiation and ongoing fluid retention throughout the breast tissue. Additionally, I continue to have a sore spot on the outside right breast. Dr. Panwalkar stated he knew how challenging it would be for me to get through the mammogram scheduled on July 25 with multiple compressions of the left breast.

Dr. Panwalkar and all of my physicians, nurses, and medical team are highly compassionate people, just as you would hope they would be when you are their patient. I reassured him I would persevere and I planned to take extra pain medication on that day prior to and following the mammogram because I knew the importance of completing the procedure. All in all, he felt I was doing as well as could be expected, considering what I had endured through my formal treatments.

After waiting almost two years for an eye exam, mostly because a number of my breast cancer-fighting medications caused blurry vision, I saw Dr. Kevin Melicher for an eye appointment on July 17. Dr. Melicher has also been going through a cancer battle, so we visited that day about a number of things we had gone through and to reassure each other we were going to be the victors in our battles. I am now set for a year with contact lenses and new lenses in my glasses, and it is a joy to be seeing better. Thank you, Dr. Melicher. You and your family will continue to be in my prayers.

Jill and I traveled to Cando on July 19 to prepare for the Impact-Cando Connection Golf Tournament, which we were hosting, along with Rusty, our other fund advisory board member, on July 21 at the Cando Golf Course. Several people volunteered to help us during the event, and we are grateful to them for sharing their time and talent. I am happy to report that we had twenty-one hole sponsors, fourteen teams, and nearly seventy people for the dinner following the golf tournament.

All proceeds and charitable gifts from this event benefit the Impact-Cando Connection Fund and will ultimately be granted back to Cando area nonprofit organizations to positively impact our hometown area. To all who participated in whatever capacity, thank you so much for helping to make this a successful and rewarding day.

I posted a photo on the website of Rusty and me at the registration table during the tournament. It was a victory for me just to get through all of the preparation and events for this day. I treasured making the milestone because I was grateful to be well enough to be there, and I quite simply love to give back to an area that has been solidly by my side through my breast cancer battle. Thank you!

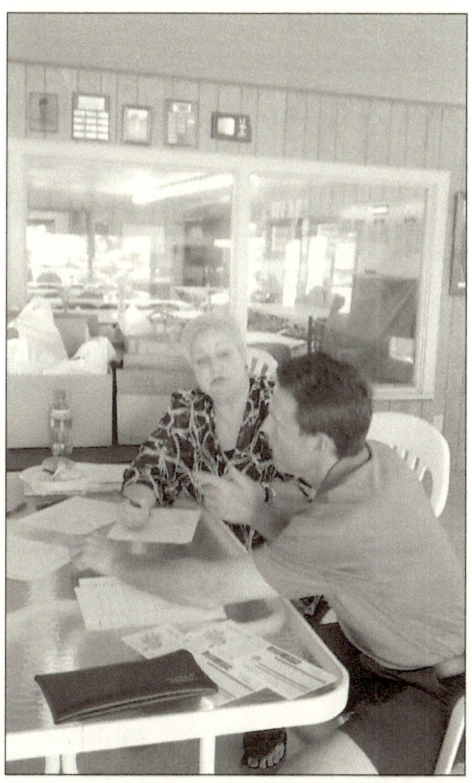

Rusty and Cindy at the registration table during the 2012 Impact-Cando Connection Golf Tournament. Another successful year ... in more ways than one!

On July 25, I completed a blood draw to check my thyroid levels (which came back at 1.9, a great test result) and the next mammogram on my left breast. Extra pain medication and sheer will got me through that procedure. The technician was absolutely wonderful. She was a blessing.

I had an appointment on July 27 with Dr. Foster to discuss my mammogram results. During the exam, he asked if the special cream I had been using for my breast pain had helped. I indicated it had reduced the overall pain, but I still had continued pain and, at times, areas in the left breast with sharp pain. I told him I understood it might just be something I had to deal with, but the cream had certainly made me feel more comfortable and better able to cope on a daily basis. Dr. Foster asked me to complete a mammogram on the right breast to once again look at the area where I have had a sore spot and have been experiencing ongoing pain since early 2011. His staff helped schedule a mammogram on my right breast for August 3.

On July 31, Dr. David Flach, my dermatologist, skillfully removed my tattoo at the base of my neck, one of three applied prior to my radiation treatments. Two of the three tattoos decided to spread, so it looked like I had a blue ink spot on my neck, and it was a constant reminder of my breast cancer battle, no matter what neckline I chose to wear. Because the tattoo had penetrated into the tissue below, Dr. Flach had to cut out some tissue, as well as remove the affected skin, and I will sport several stitches until August 14 when I return to have them removed. You don't really get a road map as to the best way to handle things like this, so you make the best decisions for yourself and go from there. God willing, I will have a small scar that will fade over time.

On August 2, I had an appointment with Dr. Hallanger-Johnson to discuss my thyroid test results and how to get me back on my feet so I could make an effort to get some weight off and slowly incorporate some exercise back into my life. With the ongoing breast pain, overall inflammation, muscle spasms, very achy knees, lightheadedness, balance issues, and sporadic nausea, every day is challenging. After talking about the difficulty in walking stairs and distances and even trying to lightly exercise, I did have X-rays of both knees completed on August 2 at Dr. Hallanger-Johnson's request to see if any deterioration needed to be addressed. I am awaiting the results.

I also told Dr. Hallanger-Johnson about episodes of not being able to think, form sentences, type, or hold a pen and feeling dizzy, so she asked me to have a brain MRI to make certain nothing else is going on health wise. It is rather disconcerting when these events happen. I try to rationalize that, because of my medications, peripheral neuropathy, chemo treatments, fatigue, and such, I should not panic and just focus on getting through the episode. However, out of precaution and at her request, I will have the brain MRI on Tuesday, August 7.

A bright spot I was able to share with her was that my tongue was almost completed healed after being diagnosed with medial rhomboid glassitis several months back. Over the past two months, I have incorporated a mega dose of vitamin B12 into my diet, and it seems to have done the trick. Another small victory!

On August 3, I completed the mammogram on my right breast, and I was asked to wait while the scans were being read. After about twenty minutes, the technician asked me to follow her back into the exam room because the doctor reading the scan wanted to speak with me. She voiced her opinion that we should complete an MRI of the right breast to get a definite answer on whether I had an ongoing issue that could not be seen because of my breast tissue being so heavy and dense. So I am also waiting for this procedure to be scheduled.

I would like to reiterate that I feel like I have been one of the more fortunate people going through a breast cancer battle. What is blatantly obvious is that you are never really done with your fight.

There is vigilant monitoring for the time being every three months and follow-up procedures, exams, blood work, and so forth as you wait with concern for the results. And even as you complete all of the overall health appointments, you still need to maintain your dental and vision health. Both are pushed aside until your schedule allows or your health stabilizes. I am still taking it one thing at a time.

I visited on July 27 with a former co-worker, back in North Dakota for a trip, who endured her own breast cancer battle about a year prior to me being diagnosed, and our conversation was enlightening. We acknowledged how similar our breast cancer battles were and the trials and tribulations of trying to recapture our lives following all the medical treatments. Thanks, Joan, for taking time to stop by and visit. You looked great and made me feel like I would make it back eventually.

I have continued to work full time, promising myself that I will listen to my doctors, nurses, and loved ones about working only an eight-hour day and then resting as much as possible before and after work. For those of you who know me well, this is as much a penance as I can imagine. I don't sit still and rest very well. Even though my body is resting, my mind certainly is not. It is screaming at me, "There is X, Y, and Z to be completed, and it won't get done with you sitting there." For those of you who have talked to me about meditation, I have been using that technique for many months to control stress, but being wired the way I am, being forced to make a change in how I live my life, has been one of the most challenging things I have ever had to do. My perspective on life and my empathy for others dealing with similar circumstances has changed dramatically.

When you want to tackle a task but physically cannot, you feel trapped, not only physically but mentally as well. Trust me. A whole lot of positive talking is happening in my head. I tell myself that the time will come soon when I can:

- Complete the chore I want to accomplish

- Take several hours to leisurely stroll, shop, and pick up items before fatigue sets in and I have to go home and rest

- Play a round of eighteen holes of golf and not ache all over for the next week

God forbid I should stop at nine holes. Call it the competitor in me. I still have visions of getting my physical, mental, and emotional self back eventually. I recognize that my spiritual self has carried me through all of the troubling news and multiple hurdles during this battle, and my same spiritual self will rejoice when the battle is truly won, when my life becomes calmer once again.

I recognize and thank each and every one of you who continue to offer up prayers, call to check on me, send an e-mail just to let me know you are thinking of me, send a card to encourage me along, and pick me up when I receive news that is not always good. Am I grateful to God for his healing, carrying me along, and blessing me on this journey? Most definitely. Do I treasure all of you for all your kindnesses? There is no doubt. Thank you! To close, I try to remember these words I read in a recent spiritual passage:

> *Our trials are great opportunities, but all too often we simply see them as large obstacles. If only we would recognize every difficult situation as something God has chosen to prove his love to us, each obstacle would then become a place of shelter and rest, and a demonstration to others of his inexpressible power. We must trust the Lord through the darkness, and honor Him with unwavering confidence even in the midst of difficult situations.* Excerpt from "Streams in the Desert" by L.B. Cowman.

Love you.

Monday, September 3, 2012, 7:30 a.m., CDT

Rebuilding My Confidence

Once we learn to wait for the Lord's leading in everything, we will know the strength that finds its highest point in an even and steady walk. Most of us are lacking the strength we so desire, but God gives complete power for every task. He calls us to perform. Waiting—keeping yourself faithful to His leading—this is the secret of strength. Excerpt from "Streams in the Desert" by L.B. Cowman.

I woke up this Labor Day morning, thanking God for the beautiful day and asking for his blessing as I wait for answers to recent medical tests I have completed. And while I wait, I continue to slowly but surely rebuild my confidence. I am capable for the most part of thinking, moving, and living my life, albeit not at the pace I used to live. But I also wait for answers to those tests that will help me rebuild my confidence, away from the constant worry of what else might be happening within my body.

On August 13, I completed the right breast MRI that Dr. Foster ordered, and I am thrilled to report that the test came back as clear. This is one of the most definitive tests that can be completed to look at the blood flow, tissue, and overall integrity of the breast, so I have felt incredibly relieved following the call from my doctor's office.

Earlier in my breast cancer battle, I was not able to complete this test in Fargo, so I always had a hint of doubt in my mind that the right breast was cancer free because I have continued to have sharp, shooting pain in that breast; however, the imaging department changed out some of their equipment so I was able to get through the test on August 13. Some great news for me following many prayers and a little more of my confidence rebuilt!

I still have several other medical issues and tests that need to be discussed and resolved. My recent brain MRI did not come back all clear, so I have an appointment with Neurology scheduled for October 16. I hope it is nothing too challenging, just aging and some side effects of my breast cancer battle and medications.

My recent X-rays of both knees show some deterioration in the right knee and an area of concern on the left knee. This is the first time in my life that I have had any knee or bone issues. It is still challenging for me to walk distances and stairs without considerable pain. I will find out more when I see the orthopedic specialist on September 11. Continuing muscle spasms are currently being treated with muscle relaxers, as necessary, and ongoing left breast pain with specially mixed cream. Hopefully, all of these issues will be resolved over time.

I know I just need to be patient, a point that my medical team hammered home, and give my body time to heal. I don't know if I ever really comprehended what I went through during my formal treatments, especially through the sixteen chemo treatments, but I have been reminded that it will take time to fully recover and I need to respect the fact my body will dictate how well I can cope from day to day.

Articles I have read, people I have spoken with who have made it through their breast cancer battles, and my medical team all have indicated it can take months, if not years, to finally feel more stable, to rebuild your confidence. So I continue to take it one day at a time, and thank God each day for his blessings and mercy. A spiritual verse I read recently really spoke to me and my situation.

Must life be considered a failure for someone compelled to stand still, forced into inaction and required to watch the great, roaring tides of life from shore? No—victory is then to be won by standing still and quietly waiting. Yet this is a thousand times harder to do than in the past, when you rushed headlong into the busyness of life. It requires much more courage to stand and wait and still not lose heart or lose hope, to submit to the will of God, to give up opportunities for work and leave honor to others, and to be quiet, confident, and rejoicing while the busy multitude goes happily along their way. Excerpt from "Streams in the Desert" by L.B. Cowman.

And yet another reading has given me hope and healing:

Blessed are those who have not seen, and yet have believed. Excerpt from "Streams in the Desert" by L.B. Cowman.

Thank you for all of your prayers, concern, e-mails, cards, and love. It is comforting knowing you have walked by my side during this long and drawn out journey. I never know what my life is going to hold, so I try to make the best of each day - knowing I would not be where I am today were it not for all of your prayers and encouragement, boundless blessings and God's grace. Take care, always! Love you.

Epilogue

I submitted the following article to the local newspaper for inclusion in a story being written about physical scars that tell a story. God once again guided me to a blank page and allowed me to write this piece, portions of which were published recently.

Physical Scars That Tell a Story

At the age of fifty-four, when I look at the scars that cover my body, I feel blessed because they are physical reminders of how fortunate I have been and how vigilant I must be to prevent scars in the future. God willing!

I have two scars on my abdomen, caused by hernia surgeries as a young girl, one completed in fourth grade and the other in sixth grade. I have a round, pink scar high on my left arm that resulted from a last-ditch attempt to make certain I was vaccinated for school. Initially, it looked like someone had burned me with a cigar, and I can't begin to tell you how many times I was asked what had caused the scar. It has paled and reduced in size over time, so it is less noticeable now.

I managed to get through high school and into my mid-forties before adding a new scar on my body. Basal cell carcinoma (skin cancer) was removed from the left side of my nose through a Mohs procedure that left a large hole down to the cartilage, which was repaired through three nose surgeries. Most people don't notice, but I do every day as I look in the mirror and thank God that a talented dermatologist was able to recognize and remove the cancer and a skilled surgeon was able to rebuild my nose over a two-year period. Taking photos was traumatic for a number of years, but I have learned to be grateful for the scar that serves as a constant reminder to schedule and complete my annual dermatology appointment where a skin scan is completed to make certain no further skin cancer has appeared.

Two scars on my back, one on my lower back and one on my left shoulder blade, continue to fade. Both represent removal of painful cysts. Neither was malignant, for which I continue to be grateful.

Three more scars were incurred in May and June 2011 when I was diagnosed with stage II breast cancer. Removal of two lumps from my left breast and nine lymph nodes from underneath my left arm were completed in a surgery in early May 2011. Another scar on my right chest was added when a port was implanted in early June 2011 so I could get through sixteen chemo treatments. The port was removed in October 2011, but it has left a sizeable, raised pink scar that will hopefully fade over time.

My most recent scar is from the removal of a blue tattoo placed high near my left collarbone prior to the thirty-three daily radiation treatments I endured for breast cancer and completed on December 30, 2011. Permanent tattoos are applied so they can be used to align the patient during radiation treatments. Some patients have small dots, the size of a pinhead, but my tattoos decided to spread so they looked like blue dots the size of a pencil eraser. So on July 31, 2012, my dermatologist removed the one tattoo that was most visible. My stitches were just removed August 14, and the nurse and a few others who have seen the incision think it will heal nicely. My prognosis following my breast cancer battle is positive, but I am also keenly aware how important staying positive and completing monthly self-breast exams, suggested mammograms, periodic checkups, and other tests are to me staying healthy. My newest scars remind me of my breast cancer journey and keep me focused.

Each of my scars has left me with a feeling that I am a better person for having them on my body. They have been character builders and remind me to be grateful and to thank God for his blessings every day.

www.ingramcontent.com/pod-product-compliance
Lightning Source LLC
Chambersburg PA
CBHW020415290526
45785CB00002B/568